Promises Kept

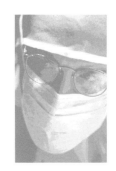

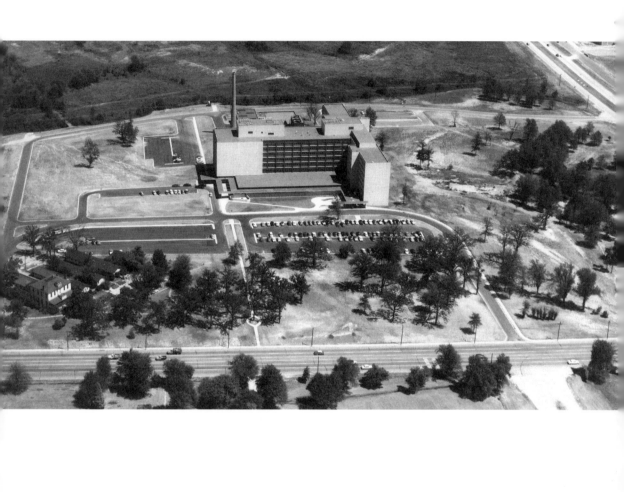

Promises Kept

The University of Mississippi Medical Center

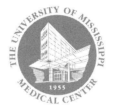

Janis Quinn

PUBLISHED BY UNIVERSITY OF MISSISSIPPI MEDICAL CENTER

DISTRIBUTED BY UNIVERSITY PRESS OF MISSISSIPPI

www.upress.state.ms.us

The University Press of Mississippi is a member of the Association of
American University Presses.

First edition 2005

∞ The paper used in this publication meets the minimum requirements of
American National Standard for Information Sciences—Permanence of Paper
for Printed Library Materials, ANSI Z39.48–1984.

Library of Congress Cataloging-in-Publication Data
Quinn, Janis.
Promises kept : the University of Mississippi Medical Center / Janis Quinn.— 1st ed.
p. ; cm.
Includes bibliographical references and index.
ISBN 1-57806-805-3 (cloth : alk. paper) 1. University of Mississippi. Medical Center—History. 2.
Medical colleges—Mississippi—History—20th century, 3. Medical education—Mississippi—His-
tory--20th century.
[DNLM: 1. University of Mississippi. Medical Center. 2. Schools, Medical—history—Mississippi.
3. Education, Medical—history—Mississippi. 4. History, 20th Century—Mississippi. W 19 Q7p
2005] I. University of Mississippi. Medical Center. II. Title.
R747.U68345Q56 2005
610'.71'1762—dc22
2005009960

British Library Cataloging-in-Publication Data available

*This history is dedicated to the Medical Center's "first family" —
those who were here first and built the very solid foundation on which all
subsequent excellence has depended.*

Contents

Acknowledgments

I would like to acknowledge all the people who so graciously gave me their time and assistance in researching and writing this history. Stan Galicki at Millsaps was generous with both his time and information about the geological history of the area. Maurine Twiss, the institution's first public information officer, provided invaluable insight into the beginning years of the Medical Center and especially the decade of the 1960s. Her unpublished history of the dental school, a valuable resource, was to be the first installment on her history of the Medical Center, a job I inherited when her health status prevented her from completing the project. She hired me in 1974 with a guarded optimism about my future there.

I am deeply indebted to Barbara Austin, Maurine Twiss's successor, Dr. Wallace Conerly, Medical Center vice chancellor from 1994 to 2003, and Dr. Dan Jones, current Medical Center vice chancellor, for their faith in my ability to write the Medical Center's story at this pivotal point in its history. I have appreciated their encouragement and assistance. Dr. Julius Cruse, the Medical Center's first Distinguished Professor of the History of Medicine, was kind enough to read the early chapters, and his reassurance saved me from overwhelming self-doubt.

Ada Seltzer, Rowland Medical Library director, gave me a station in the archives so that I could easily access and use archival information. David Juergens was most helpful in negotiating the archival information.

Anne Graeber took me to heretofore unknown closets to locate files from the Norman C. Nelson years and fought a decade's collection of dust and insects to help me retrieve boxes and haul them to the archives.

I love the Medical Center. I have loved it since 1974 when I walked up the hill from the stadium on a hot July afternoon to be interviewed by Maurine Twiss. I was captivated thirty years ago by the same sense of purpose and dedication that caught the attention of the University of Mississippi chancellor Robert Khayat. When he first became chancellor, he came to the Medical Center every Thursday for touring and teaching sessions with then vice chancellor Dr. Wallace Conerly. He told me that while he was still learning his way around the Medical Center and learning how things fit together, he was struck by what he called "the wonderful spirit of this place." And while it is true that the center has been the beneficiary of gifted leaders in its fifty-year history, it has also reaped the rewards of having a committed work force, people who somehow "buy into" the mission of the Medical Center and do their utmost to carry it out. They make the Medical Center what it is. They are its "wonderful spirit." To all of them, "Thank you."

Promises Kept

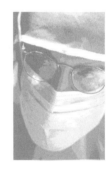

CHAPTER 1

Our Island Home

The University of Mississippi Medical Center occupies 164 acres approximately two miles north of downtown Jackson in Hinds County, in the geographic center of Mississippi. This history will deal primarily with the people who have shaped and molded the original two-year medical school at the University of Mississippi in Oxford and later, the University of Mississippi Medical Center in Jackson. But the land on which it stands has its own history, and true to our heritage as southerners, no history is complete without a nod to the forces that shaped the land before it came to us.

Long before there was a Jackson, long before there was a United States, even before the appearance of man on the earth, the home of the Medical Center was part of a small island in a tropical sea. Some 79 million years ago, the island stretched across about 185 square miles—an area that extended as far west as what is now Clinton in Hinds County, as far east as Brandon's western city limits in Rankin County, as far north as the southern limits of Ridgeland in Madison County, and as far south as the southern limits of Richland, also in Rankin County. Our island home rose from the sea as a result of volcanic eruptions, which also pushed up the layers of sediment, which had lain under the shallow sea. With the cone of the volcano located some 2,600 feet below what is now the Jackson Coliseum, the volcanic push distributed the upended sediment in a circle around the area.

Geologists call this sediment from this ancient sea the Yazoo clay of the Jackson Group. These ancient events are pertinent to the story of the Medical Center, because, like many homeowners in the area where Yazoo clay is near the surface, Medical Center administrators and engineers have long grappled with the destructive forces of this ancient goo. When the clay is wet, it expands. In hot, dry months, the clay dries and contracts. The movement caused by the shrinking and expanding can literally tear a house apart, causing masonry to crack, windows to lose their frames, and floors to slope.

The Jackson Dome, the geological name for the area formed by the ancient volcano, the area that was the island, is also the place where the Yazoo clay is nearest the surface and therefore problematic to foundations.

The band of Yazoo clay actually stretches from Yazoo County to the west and eastward to Clarke and Wayne counties. The clay farthest from the dome is also farthest from the surface and, therefore, presents few problems for construction. The average thickness of the band of clay around the Jackson Dome is 450 feet. The 30 or so feet of clay nearest the surface is subject to the vagaries of the weather, so builders who take the clay into account dig beyond the 30 feet and sink foundation supports into the clay that is unaffected by water and drought on the surface.

As early as 1960, the Medical Center's power plant was the first victim of the clay's destructive force. Billy Williams, who retired as assistant director of physical facilities in 2001, recalled that the Yazoo clay had moved the slab in the power plant and that had destroyed the electric feeders, which then had to be replaced.

In 1990, the Medical Center's physical plant director at the time, Glenn Ray, estimated that repairing damage to the west wing of University Hospital would cost $700,000. The foundation of one of the original hospital wings had shifted so severely, the basement was of practically no use for offices. Office chairs would roll down the slope of the basement floor. Subsequent construction plans on campus have factored in the Yazoo clay by deep excavation, backfilling, and leaving a space to allow the clay freedom of movement.

In later geologic periods, Jackson would be covered by water again, waters would recede, the dinosaurs would disappear, and mammals would emerge as the dominant life force. Sometimes, it is only the clay, rich with fossil remains, that reminds us of earlier inhabitants. Measured in geologic time, human occupancy of the 164 acres is as brief as an eye blink. "Prehistory" was yesterday.

The city of Jackson was settled a few years after Mississippi entered the union in 1817. Originally owned by the Choctaw Indians, it was ceded to the federal government by the Treaty of Doaks Stand in 1820. Jackson was incorporated in 1823.

The site of the present University of Mississippi Medical Center was the home of the State Insane Hospital, which accepted its first patients on January 8, 1855, one hundred years before the University Hospital accepted its first patients in July 1955.

The hospital for the insane, alternately called the state insane asylum and the state lunatic asylum, was the fifth major public building erected in the growing state capital.

Its construction was preceded by the first statehouse, on the corner of Capitol and President streets, completed in 1822; the second statehouse, which now houses the Old Capitol Museum on State Street, completed in 1839; the present-day governor's mansion, completed in 1842; and the penitentiary, on land bordered by President, West, Mississippi, and High streets, completed in 1840.

In 1848, in a move that coincided with the era of reform in the rest of the country, the Mississippi Legislature authorized the establishment of a "lunatic asylum" in Jackson. A similar bill in 1846 was defeated. The city appropriated five acres for the purpose, and the legislature made $10,000 available for the building and directed the state prison to have inmates make the bricks. The five commissioners appointed to oversee the building and operation of the asylum sold the five acres given by the city for $700 and bought another 140 acres for $1,750. That 140 acres is included in the present-day 164-acre tract. Another act of the legislature in 1848 changed the name from lunatic asylum to Insane Hospital.

The mid-nineteenth century in American history was a time of social reform. The causes of women's suffrage, public education, the abolition of slavery, and the humane treatment of prisoners and the insane were each taken on by individuals and groups committed to a new order of moral responsibility. Among those reformers was Dorothea Dix, a Boston schoolteacher who was the most active advocate of state-supported mental hospitals. The noted crusader made a trip to Jackson in 1850 to further the cause of the state's asylum. The 1850s was also the time of great prosperity for the state. Major cotton production shifted from the Southeast into the Alabama-Mississippi Black Belt and the Mississippi Delta. The state had the money it needed for the asylum.

After many delays in construction, including a completely new start, the asylum was finished seven years after it was authorized. Present-day Medical Center administrators, often faced with delays in construction, could find solace in the history of the asylum's construction. Innumerable delays were attributed to high water on the Pearl River, low water on the Ohio River, yellow fever epidemics, unfavorable weather at the building site, and failure of the penitentiary to deliver the bricks promptly.

In 1848, Governor Joseph W. Matthews appointed Dr. William S. Langley, Thomas J. Catchings, William Morris, H. Hilzheim, and C. S. Tarpley as the first commissioners to oversee the asylum's construction. They hired William Gibbons as the architect.

Gibbons reported to the legislature in 1850 that the walls of the first story were almost complete, and approximately 800,000 bricks laid. But Gibbons was not to finish the project. That same year, Gov. John A. Quitman appointed F. S. Hunt, C. H. Manship, and J. H. Boyd and renewed the appointments of Dr. William S. Langley and C. S. Tarpley as commissioners. (Langley became the first superintendent of the asylum.) This group of commissioners hired another architect, Joseph Willis, who expressed grave concerns about the newly constructed foundation for the asylum.

As a result, a team of independent inspectors declared the foundation unsafe, the first walls were demolished, and the whole project started anew. In a lengthy report to commissioners, Willis says that he was of the opinion "that it would be better to take up all the walls, but in order to save as much as possible, I thought we could secure the building by making all the outside and main cross walls substantial." But the inspectors confirmed that "the walls and foundations were incompetent to sustain the superstructure that was intended to be put upon them."

In rebuilding the foundation, Willis encountered what countless construction crews at the Medical Center have found since—a reminder of the ancient volcano.

> I found, that in excavating the cellar that all the clay had been removed, and that the walls had been built on a bed of marl, that extends to the depth of from twenty to thirty feet, and that when it is wet, expands and becomes soft and slippery, and that when dry, it contracts and becomes hard, and if exposed to the atmosphere, crumbles or slacks like lime; consequently, it is a very poor material for foundations for buildings. In fact, from what little experience I have had in this kind of earth, I am satisfied that here must be some kind of an artificial foundation created to build upon, in order to sustain a building of any magnitude.

The original asylum building accommodated 160 patients. Between 1890 and 1891 two brick wings were added—one for black males and one for black females. At the end of 1891, the asylum had 471 patients. To serve the needs of patients who also suffered from a medical illness, a new hospital was added between 1911 and 1913 with a 100-bed capacity.

The superintendent appointed in 1918, Dr. Charles D. Mitchell, served the next sixteen years without interruption. It was Mitchell who recommended that a new hospital be built in Rankin County following the modern trend of cottage housing. In the Biennial Report of 1923–1925 he noted that "there has not been a single room added for the past 14 years and before Jan. 1 (1926) we will have 2000 patients and the limit will have been reached." The legislature appropriated $2.5 million in 1926 for a new hospital, and the present Mississippi State Hospital at Whitfield opened in 1935.

During its eighty years on the site in Jackson, the asylum staff took care of thousands of people. Many of the patients had transient illnesses and were discharged. For others it was their last refuge. When they died, their bodies were either claimed by their relatives and buried with other family members, or sadly, unclaimed and buried on asylum grounds.

In the Biennial Report for 1900–1901, the asylum reported the cost of fifty-four coffins in 1900 and fifty-six in 1901. It seems logical that these coffins were for inmates whose bodies were unclaimed and who were buried on asylum property. And if years preceding and following 1900 and 1901 recorded similar numbers of coffins purchased, then it's possible that some hundreds of inmates were buried on the grounds of the asylum. Some of these graves would surface in 1992 during the laying of pipe for the construction of the Medical Center's new laundry.

Marked graves were present when the governor deeded the land to the University of Mississippi in 1960, but by that time, many had been vandalized and some of the gravestones removed. There has been some conflict, over the years, between historical preservationists and Medical Center administrators who often disagreed over the fate of the buried remains. Who could blame either side, really? On the one hand, Medical Center leaders were always looking for the least costly way to expand the center's physical plant in the face of growing demands of health education and health care. On the other hand, equally committed historians were seeking to preserve a vital link to our past.

In 1973, the legislature gave the Medical Center permission to rebury any remains it found in the course of excavating for construction. In 1992, while digging a large ditch for a steam line that would connect the new laundry with the power plant, a construction crew began to uncover wooden boxes that could only be coffins and the skeletal remains therein. (The old laundry had been another casualty of Yazoo clay. Built as part of the original complex, the building's shifting foundation had caused such destruction that the building had been declared unsafe.)

Before the ditch was completed, a total of forty-four graves were uncovered. In accordance with the 1973 statute, Dr. Wallace Conerly (vice chancellor from 1994 to 2003) ordered the remains reburied. He directed the physical facilities staff to create the Asylum Cemetery. The remaining marked graves and their stones, together with the unmarked graves uncovered during the laundry excavation, were buried there. Dr. Ruth Black, hospital chaplain and director of pastoral services, officiated at a formal ceremony consecrating the new burial ground in 1994. The unmarked graves lie under a marker listing all the names of those known to have been buried on asylum grounds, and "to those unknown." The cemetery now serves as the repository for the ashes of those who donate their bodies for anatomical dissection. The health professional students who have used the bodies in gross anatomy speak at an annual ceremony at the cemetery honoring the donors. The cremated remains of infants and stillborns, also buried in the cemetery at the parents' request, are recognized and memorialized in another annual service called the Ceremony of Remembrance.

The asylum grounds had a cameo appearance in the Civil War and left present-day inhabitants with another permanent reminder of the land's past. Federal forces under the command of Brig. Gen. Thomas Welsh occupied the asylum grounds and flew the colors of the Forty-fifth Pennsylvania from the asylum's cupola. According to Edwin C. Bearss in *The Siege of Jackson*, "As Union skirmishers pursued retreating butternuts across the asylum's spacious grounds, some of the 150 inmates rushed to the windows and shouted excitedly at the troops. Fortunately, none of these people was hurt, though several minie balls struck the building." When federal forces occupied Jackson, they erected earthworks at strategic points for firing on Confederate troops. One of these formations remains on the grounds near the School of Dentistry.

Sometime between the asylum's opening and 1900, the legislature gave the asylum additional land, and at one time, the land area occupied by the asylum totaled more than thirteen hundred acres. The acreage was necessary for the asylum's vast farming enterprise that supplied food for inmates and to sell to the community. The inmates ate well, benefiting from the harvest of their own pecan and fruit orchards and strawberry fields. They grew corn and hay, cabbage, turnips, tomatoes, and potatoes and "all vegetables grown in the South have been furnished the patients in abundance." Thirty-five acres were devoted to truck farming in 1900, and the asylum staff raised 450 hogs. In the Biennial Report of 1900–1901, the administration reported that raising hogs cost nothing but the original price and performed a valuable service (in addition to the meat) in consuming "the immense amount of kitchen slop that accumulates."

The asylum lands also became the subject of a legal dispute during the state's first foray into oil and gas drilling. As the ancient volcano became dormant, erosion of the volcanic island caused a reef to form around it. This reef, geologists predicted, would produce copious amounts of gas and oil. In 1924, the asylum's board of trustees granted Ella Rawls Reader Stokely a lease on the asylum lands to drill for gas. She began drilling in 1925 near the present site of the Smith-Wills Stadium and the Agricultural Museum grounds—land that no longer belongs to the university. She drilled through gas that was later discovered, but her wells never produced. The state contended that the board of trustees had no authority to grant the lease, and in 1934, a federal court concurred, and she lost the lease. Now the state was in the oil business with the State Mineral Lease Commission, and for a sum of $115,000 appropriated by the legislature, drilling began again on the asylum property. The first state well blew up, leaving a crater twenty yards across. As Dudley J. Hughes describes it in his book, *Oil in the Deep South: A History of the Oil Business in Mississippi, Alabama, and Florida, 1859–1945*:

On that fateful day, Henry M. Kendall, a young Jackson attorney, was returning from a squirrel hunt on horseback through what is now Riverside Park. As he approached the state's drilling rig, it suddenly exploded. Drillpipe shot into the air with a cloud of mud, rocks and other debris. The wooden derrick began disintegrating and the crew members ran for their lives. The roar was deafening. Soon a crater erupted like a volcano a short distance away from the rig and swallowed one of the boilers. The next day the blowout killed itself, the crater then filling with water and mud.

After the move to Rankin County in 1935, the old asylum grounds stood vacant for many years. And while asylum officials were busy reorganizing in their new location, the medical school at the University of Mississippi in Oxford was in the throes of a crisis that led inexorably to the establishment of the University of Mississippi Medical Center in Jackson in 1955 on the same land that had been in the state's hands for more than a century.

CHAPTER 2

Bilbo Medicine, Guyton Healing

Alfred Benjamin Butts, named chancellor of the University of Mississippi in 1935, began his tenure as the state and the university struggled to recover from the ravages of the Great Depression. David Sansing, author of *The University of Mississippi: A Sesquicentennial History*, calls Butts the university's "best educated and most visionary chancellor since Frederick Barnard."

Sansing also called Butts's appointment of Dr. Billy Sylvester Guyton as dean of the medical school one of the chancellor's "most notable achievements."

A 1911 graduate of the university's medical school, Guyton was a successful ophthalmologist in Oxford and part-time teacher at the school in 1935 when he agreed to serve one year as acting dean. When that year was up, he told Butts he would stay until the job was finished. What Guyton accomplished as dean during that critical decade of the 1930s was, quite simply, the school's survival.

Guyton's reluctance to accept the deanship is easily understood in light of what he was agreeing to: leadership of a school plagued by political interference, facing the bleakest financial period in the state's bleak financial history, and threatened with the loss of accreditation and closure. Guyton also very likely understood what Sansing has noted: "While it may not be that Billy Guyton can be solely credited with saving the medical school, it is safe to assume that if it failed, he would certainly have gotten most of the blame."

This small two-year program in rural Mississippi is the foundation of the University of Mississippi Medical Center—a major academic health sciences campus with five schools and four hospitals. Had the medical school in Oxford not won its struggle for survival in the 1930s, the Medical Center would not exist as we know it today. Establishing a four-year school from zero, without the base of the two-year school, would have been much more difficult and would have taken years longer.

The medical school in Oxford began as the Department of Medicine in 1903. In this two-year program, its graduates completed courses in basic sciences—anatomy, physical chemistry (later biochemistry), bacteriology (later named microbiology), pharmacology, and physiology. They went on to schools that had full four-year programs with teaching hospitals for their last two years. From 1911 until 1955, 124 two-year graduates went on to posts in academic medicine. This is just one way to measure the quality of an educational program, and it showed that the medical school ranked favorably with other institutions, private and public. One of its more famous graduates was Dr. Thomas F. Frist (certificate, 1931), who taught at Vanderbilt and founded the giant Hospital Corporation of America (HCA), later changed to Quorum Health Services, one of the nation's largest health care corporations.

The two-year curriculum was a common configuration for medical education in the early years of the twentieth century, but it was coming under increased criticism in the 1930s.

According to Lucie Bridgforth in *Medical Education in Mississippi: A History of the School of Medicine*, sixteen students enrolled in 1903 under what would be considered very lax admission standards one hundred years later. They had to be sixteen, provide certificates attesting to their good moral character, and bring with them records of successful work in either college, normal school, or high school. But just as the two-year medical school was the norm in the United States, so were the undemanding entrance requirements. It would be decades before medicine became the highly competitive curriculum with its exacting entrance requirements that it is today.

The school fared well when the Carnegie Foundation published Abraham Flexner's exhaustive report on the status of medical education in the United States in 1910. Flexner, whose ideal in medical education was Johns Hopkins in Baltimore (established in 1893), didn't exactly give Mississippi's school a resounding affirmation, but did call it "distinctly creditable." Although one of Flexner's great ideals in medical education was that a medical school be affiliated with a university, his twin ideal was adequate clinical training in a hospital, and he said that the university was "unfortunately located" for such a purpose.

The Flexner Report, the first-ever report on the status of medical education in the United States to name names and schools, effectively closed many of the so-called proprietary medical schools that had proliferated in the second half of the nineteenth century. Mississippi had at least one—the Meridian Medical College in Meridian owned by a group of physicians. Illinois at the same time had thirty-nine such schools. The schools, lacking any university oversight and no uniform standards, had produced a glut of physicians who were poorly trained. Flexner's goal was to have fewer, better-trained physicians. Even though Flexner was not overly enthusiastic about the University's school in Mississippi, he perhaps saw it as the only alternative for a poor state to educate its citizens in the practice of medicine.

After the report, the school was in good standing with the two agencies it looked to for accreditation until 1927 when the Association of American Medical Colleges (AAMC) placed the school on probation. The association cited an inadequate budget, too few faculty, and poor facilities. Although the school's plight during the 1930s is often laid at the feet of Governor Theodore Bilbo, the school's probationary status came three years before Bilbo fired the university chancellor, Dr. Alfred Hume, and the dean of the medical school, Dr. Joseph Crider, during what is often referred to as the "Bilbo purge." The populist governor saw himself as an educational reformer and tried single-handedly to improve higher education in Mississippi. He selectively fired and hired college presidents, deans, and faculty members. Bilbo fired Crider precisely because the AAMC had put the school on probation under Crider's watch, and Bilbo held Crider responsible. Ironically, Bilbo's firing of Crider brought the school under closer scrutiny by the accrediting agencies. The agencies didn't care how pure Bilbo's motives might have been; what concerned them most was the degree to which an elected official could control what should be left in the hands of educators.

Bilbo's actions brought the national spotlight to higher education in the state, and the bright light illuminated inadequacies not easy to fix in the aftermath of the stock market crash in 1929 and the ensuing depressed economy. Even before the Great Depression of the 1930s, Mississippi's agricultural-based economy had suffered blows from a decline in the export market and from boll weevil infestations. The national depression just made a terrible situation worse.

In Bilbo's zeal to reform higher education, he wanted Mississippi to have the best in progressive education, and the University of Mississippi became a main focus. He first urged the legislature to move the University to Jackson (to the land now occupied by the University of Mississippi Medical Center), a proposal nixed by the legislature after howls of protest from Oxford. When that idea got no hearing, Bilbo asked the legislature for $5 million. He got $1.6 million to upgrade the university. This money in 1928 enabled the university to begin construction on a badly needed new building for the medical school that would house more laboratories and classrooms as well as a campus hospital. This building would not be finished until Guyton was dean, in 1937, and it was the only thing the school could point to in 1928 that it had done to meet the accreditation requirements. Failing to enthrall the legislature with his ideas for reforming higher education, Bilbo turned to the Board of Trustees of Institutions of Higher Learning (IHL), overseeers of the state's public colleges. In 1930, he made three key appointments that gave him control of the board. So, according to Bridgforth, Bilbo achieved by "executive power what he had been unable to achieve through legislative action."

Bilbo, through his handpicked board, fired Chancellor Hume and the president of Mississippi A & M (now Mississippi State University). The board also fired a number of teachers in all schools at the university, including the medical school. The outcry in the wake of such bold political interference was deafening, but Bilbo's actions were not unilaterally bad. Many of the changes he instituted were needed. The people who replaced those selected for dismissal by the governor were almost always better qualified. Contrary to popular opinion, Bilbo sometimes fired those who had supported him politically if he thought they weren't doing the job. His critics often reported that as many as seventy-three faculty members at the university had been dismissed during Bilbo's sweep, although the university administration listed only sixteen teachers whose contracts were not renewed. His imperious attitude hid his honorable intentions, and the press accounts of his actions were almost entirely negative. National media representatives called him "the Mussolini of Mississippi" and described his heavy hand in public higher education as "the spoils system."

Bilbo's firing of Dean Crider led to a warning from the AAMC and from the Council on Medical Education and Hospitals of the American Medical Association (AMA) that went well beyond probation: If Crider was not reinstated, the school would lose its A rating. The board of trustees reinstated Crider, only to be notified of his resignation two days before the beginning of the fall semester in 1930. Bilbo also fired faculty member Dr. Peter Rowland; he thought Rowland, at sixty-nine, was too old to be an effective teacher. The board never found a replacement for Rowland so he remained on the faculty despite his age. Rowland went on to leave a lasting legacy. Dr. Philip Mull, a former anatomy professor in the school, served as the next dean and oversaw the school's futile efforts to meet the demands of accreditation.

On the issue of political interference, the two agencies seemed to have been mollified by Crider's reinstatement, but they backed off again when the Southern Association of Colleges and Schools (SACS) suspended the university along with Mississippi A & M, Mississippi State College for Women (now Mississippi University for Women), and the state teachers' college in Hattiesburg (now the University of Southern Mississippi). This major accreditation body, of which the university was a charter member, dismissed the university from its ranks for what it termed "ruthless" action by the governor and the board of trustees. It would be two years before the university was back in the good graces of SACS. After an extensive evaluation, the agency agreed to reinstate the university if certain conditions were met, including the rehiring of fired chancellor Hume. Hume got his job back in 1932 and stayed until 1935.

Hume, according to Sansing, was probably the most-beloved chancellor in the history of the university. Hume and Bilbo had a basic difference of opinion about what an education should be. In Hume's view, an education should mold character and contribute to moral growth. Bilbo viewed public education as a tool to bring progress to the state. The practicality of a medical education was one reason Bilbo was so interested in the state's only medical school. He saw its value to the health of the state, a view that helped create the University of Mississippi Medical Center twenty-five years later.

With the university's membership in SACS restored, and the political storm calmed, the medical school remained under the friendly but eagle-eyed scrutiny of the AMA and the AAMC, whose leaders continued to point out the school's inadequate budget, facilities, and faculty. But it was 1932, and compliance with the demands of the two agencies would be costly. The state was cash poor. The agencies saw the need for more laboratories and better equipment, a hospital where students could see the practical application of the basic sciences they were learning in the classroom, more faculty, higher faculty salaries, and a better library. In 1932, the medical library had fewer than one thousand volumes. It needed, according to the AMA and the AAMC, an additional three thousand volumes and fifty of the leading medical journals.

In 1932, Mississippi's annual per capita income was $126. The state had the highest unemployment rate in its history; the state treasury was empty; and the state was $50 million in debt. For much of that year, in the very depths of the Great Depression, faculty went without salaries. The legislature faced these grim statistics and looked for ways to slash the budget. One way was to eliminate the medical school and the pharmacy school because they were too expensive to maintain, they said. Supporters convinced lawmakers not to close the schools, but ended with a 40 percent cut in appropriations. The AMA agreed to extend the school's probationary status until July 1, 1934, to give the school time to meet accreditation standards. The AAMC gave it until November 1, 1935. A year after the medical school fought off closure and suffered a drastic cut in appropriations, school officials were back in the legislature in 1933 asking for an emergency appropriation to prevent the AAMC and the AMA from "expelling" the school from their ranks. In March 1934, the legislature set aside $75,000 that was used to complete the medical building begun in 1929, to renovate the old medical building, and to enlarge the faculty.

The school made great strides in meeting accreditation demands with the cooperation of Dean Mull, Chancellor Hume, Governor Mike Conner, and the state legislature. The fall 1934 semester opened optimistically. But when spring came to the campus so did the site visitors from the AMA and the AAMC. The inspection team stayed on campus for three days in March 1935 as part of a nationwide tour of medical education facilities that had nothing to do with the accreditation crisis up to that point. The team's evaluation of the medical school was unfavorable even given the improvements already made or underway. University officials expressed surprise that the agencies, heretofore friendly and helpful, were showing a meaner side.

Dr. Thurman Kitchin, dean of the two-year medical school of Wake Forest College, believed that the fate of the nation's two-year schools had already been decided before the "tour" began. Kitchin's conviction was that the AMA Council had a hidden agenda to eliminate the two-year schools regardless of quality. According to Kitchin, the council feared an oversupply of physicians and saw eliminating the two-year schools as the least painful remedy.

Dean Philip Mull, in poor health and weary from the intense hardships of the last five years, resigned on June 1, 1935, three months after the last blow to the school was delivered. "We have about come to the end of our period of grace," Mull told the chancellor.

This, then, was the state of the school when Dr. Billy Guyton accepted a one-year term as acting dean of the medical school. As though state finances and political interference were not enough to overcome, Guyton now faced the possibility that the school's closure was predetermined.

The fateful visit in the spring of 1935 led to a new state of uncertainty. In a six-page letter to Dr. William Cutter, secretary of the AMA Council on Medical Education and Hospitals, Chancellor Hume wrote, "To say that his apparently unfriendly attitude struck a stunning blow is not putting it too strongly." Hume referred to comments made by Dr. H. G. Weiskotten, dean of the Syracuse University medical school, the inspector representing the AMA Council. The other inspector, representing the AAMC, was Father Alphonse M. Schwitalla. Hume's letter to Cutter offers a detailed list of excerpts from correspondence with AAMC and AMA officials that show that the two agencies gave nothing but encouragement in the university's attempt to meet accreditation requirements; that agency officials were part of the decision-making process in the renovation of the medical building and in the hiring of faculty; and that they were uniformly positive in their assessment of the university's ability to regain its A standing.

Therefore, the view of the two inspectors was, as Hume stated, "a stunning blow."

The executive secretary of the IHL board, W. H. Smith, described the state of affairs of the medical school after the inspection to board members in a memo dated March 20, 1935. "The expressions of the inspectors indicated an unfavorable attitude toward the question of approval. They reflected an unfriendly attitude toward the policy of approving two-year schools in general and especially in an institution with a strictly rural setting. They indicated that the school does not, in their judgment, meet the standard requirements and a doubt that it ever would. In view of the understanding we had with the accrediting agencies before we started on this program we were shocked to realize that our efforts and expenditures may have been in vain."

After Guyton had been in the dean's office six weeks, he pointed out two particular communications from Cutter (AMA) and Dr. Fred C. Zapffe (AAMC) to Chancellor Butts in a July 16, 1935, letter. From Cutter: "[A]t its meeting on June 9, the Council (on Medical Education and Hospitals) voted that the recent survey of the University of Mississippi School of Medicine does not justify the re-instatement of the institution as an approved school of medicine."

From Zapffe: "It might be well for you to consider securing the approval for the transfer of your students to a four-year school from the Council on Medical Education until such time as the status of the school is passed on definitely. It is my understanding that former approval expired July 1, 1934. I may be in error, but advise you look into the matter. Of course, so far as this Association is concerned, the school is on probation, therefore the students in attendance will be recognized, if the medical schools wish to take them on, but you really should have them covered by the Council as well to avoid any unpleasantness which might arise."

With two seemingly conflicting opinions from the two agencies, it was now Guyton's task to determine the true status of the school—on probation or unapproved? To understand where the school stood, Guyton asked to meet with Cutter and Zapffe, which he did on July 11, 1935. The litany of problems described by the two was the same as it had been since 1927, although Guyton noted that they did recognize the great improvements made. Cutter told him there were too few full-time faculty, the budget ($27,000) was half what it should be, and faculty salaries should be substantially higher. Physical equipment and facilities, greatly improved with the aid of the 1934 legislative appropriation, were "better than some . . . but not as good as others."

The main problem, as Guyton understood it from Cutter and Zapffe, was one in common with other two-year schools. A growing trend in medical education was earlier exposure of students to patients. To meet this requirement would mean a major reorganization of curriculum and would require the cooperation of nearby hospitals or agreements with hospitals in Jackson to allow students time in their setting. The students would also need to observe and participate in autopsies during their second year, problematic in a rural area with few hospitals. Up until this point, students did their surgical pathology training after they transferred to another, larger school with a hospital. But that, too, was being recommended during an earlier year.

Guyton told Chancellor Butts that "perhaps during the next year the Council will in all likelihood establish a definite policy toward all two-year schools. At present it appears this policy will not be favorable, although probably will not entirely abolish the schools. Almost certainly they will have to accomplish some reorganization."

The most immediate problem, Guyton pointed out to Butts, was how to assure that the students just finishing their first year be accepted for transfer at the end of their second year. These were students who enrolled as first-year students in the fall of 1934 when the outlook, from the school's vantage, was rosy. They were caught in the middle of a storm not of their making, and Guyton was determined to see that they did not suffer.

The second pressing problem was whether to admit a freshman class in the fall of 1935. One of Guyton's first decisions as dean was probably his most difficult. Even though the previous fall enrollment had been up (twenty-two in the freshman class) and there were many applicants to choose from this year, Guyton and Butts, with approval from the board, decided that the situation looked so ominous that a freshman class would not be enrolled. Now it was no longer a matter of a delay in accreditation. There was a good possibility the school would be closed permanently.

From Guyton's letters to Dr. Waller S. Leathers, the dean of the Vanderbilt University School of Medicine and first dean of the Mississippi school, there is an indication that some back-door maneuvering was indeed part of the process.

AMA's Cutter sent Guyton a telegram on September 17, 1935, to say that the council did not take any action concerning the Mississippi students, those Guyton was worried about transferring. Cutter said he would write later. In a September 27 letter Cutter reported on a resolution passed by the AMA Council at its meeting in Denver: "After July 1, 1938, the Council on Medical Education and Hospitals of the American Medical Association will not publish a list of approved two-year schools." This resolution was published in the October 5, 1935, issue of the *Journal of the American Medical Association*. Cutter also said, "The Council did not feel justified in giving its approval to the members of your second-year class at the present time, but this action does not preclude the possibility of a reconsideration based on further information as to the policy of the school."

To Leathers, Guyton wrote on November 27, 1935, "Dr. Cutter did not present our request to the Council in the Denver meeting for the transfer of our students, and yet he has indicated by telegram, letter and personal conversation that the Council considered our request and then failed to grant it."

Leathers writes back, December 4, 1935, "You must remember that you are dealing with individuals who are pretty hard-boiled and it may require some 'clubbing' to get over your point of view."

Guyton had already done some of his own "clubbing" by contacting each member of the AMA Council in advance of the December 8 meeting in Chicago with a personal request to approve the transfer of the nineteen sophomore students and to be "placed back in the class of the other two-year schools and be permitted to share with them such advantages that you are granting them until July, 1938." Guyton says in his letter he is confident the school can meet the requirements of the council. "Prominent men in all walks of life in our state are clamoring for a four-year school, but we who are connected with the State University wish only to be allowed to continue the two-year school. Such a school could not forever transfer students to approved four-year schools if the students were not well trained. The school would be forced to die for lack of getting their students accepted for junior and senior year. However, many four-year schools tell us our students do well in their institutions."

The resolution that called for the council not to include two-year schools on its approved list would have effectively closed them. In 1935, Mississippi had one of the nine 2-year schools in the country. The resolution would have closed the Wake Forest medical school, the medical school at Chapel Hill, North Carolina, Dartmouth medical school in New Hampshire, the University of Alabama medical school, and medical schools in Utah, Missouri, South Dakota, and North Dakota.

At an AAMC meeting in Toronto (October 28–30, 1935), the organization asked the AMA Council to reconsider its resolution, and passed a resolution of its own that instructed the secretary to "advise the AMA Council that the AAMC requests the Council to reconsider its action upon the two-year medical schools and to classify such schools individually on their respective merits."

Dr. William Pepper of the University of Pennsylvania offered the successful motion. He called the action of the AMA Council "rather precipitate." He also pointed out that he, like others, depended on the two-year school for a steady supply of good students. "I have personally admitted 611 students to the third-year class of our school of medicine, . . . I have studied the scholastic attainment of the students from these two-year schools, and have been in the habit each year of sending to the deans of these schools a statistical table showing how their former students have made out. The fact that I have admitted 611 shows that I appreciate the product of those schools. I want to keep on admitting them. I would very much hate to have that supply cut off." Dr. O. W. Hyman, dean of the University of Tennessee medical school, which accepted many of the Mississippi graduates, said he wanted to hear Pepper's resolution "heartily endorsed."

The council did vote to reconsider the resolution, and Cutter notified Chancellor Butts of that decision by letter on December 14, 1935. He also told Butts that the council voted that the two-year schools would be considered individually instead of collectively. By separate letter he told Butts that the sophomore class "may be accepted in approved schools without prejudice" and that the status of the Mississippi school would be deferred until the February 1936 meeting of the council.

Acting on the recommendations from that first meeting with Cutter and Zapffe, Guyton was busy making arrangements with hospitals and clinics accessible to the campus where students could get clinical experience and autopsy experience. He wrote to the deans of most of the country's four-year medical schools to get detailed reports on budgets, faculty salaries, and necessary hospital equipment to run a four-year school. He at first envisioned having the last two years of the curriculum in Jackson with the first two years remaining in Oxford. If accreditation demanded the state create a four-year curriculum, he would know what kind of resources would be required.

But in a January 15, 1936, letter to Dr. R. W. Hall, a Jackson dermatologist and member of the executive committee of the Central Medical Society, Guyton acknowledges AMA's hard line with other two-year schools and tells him plans for a four-year school now may be premature. The Jackson Chamber of Commerce as well as the medical establishment had apparently responded with some enthusiasm to the notion of having the last two years of the curriculum in Jackson. But Guyton tells Hall that the AMA Council had already put ten 4-year schools on probation and had warned five others. Many of these schools, Guyton said, "have equipment worth a million or more and some of them have been running 50 years or more." For Mississippi to start such an enterprise now, with such limited means, would doom it to failure, he believed. He tells Hall that "we have better hopes now of getting our two-year school in good standing."

Several days before the February meeting of the executive council that would decide the school's fate, Guyton wrote the AMA executive council member Weiskotten, the outspokenly critical inspector during the previous spring's visit, to explain the dilemma facing the school: The probationary status, imposed by the AMA, was keeping the school from making the changes mandated by the AMA to get its A rating back.

"When we go before our Board of Trustees and committees from the legislature in regard to the budget," Guyton wrote, "they wish to know if our school is in good standing, and if not, why not, since they have given us money for making improvements in the past few years. They wish to know also if we have any assurance that we will get back into first class standing should they grant our request and give us more liberal support. Two years ago, we asked for seventy-five thousand dollars for some improvements in one lump sum. This was given to us, and it was spent for new equipment. It was thought that this would place us in a position to expect the removal of the probation status. Now when we ask for further funds and more equipment, they cannot understand why we did not get back into good standing after the special appropriation given us at that time." He hastens to add that many members of the legislature are Ole Miss alumni and "we feel confident we shall secure a liberal appropriation for our budget this year."

Guyton also points out the record of their students when they transfer to other schools, who "ranked either in the middle or upper third of the graduating class." He notes that this standing had been maintained even through the five-year probation period. "This is true in spite of the handicap in which probation has placed us in regard to the students."

To the meeting on February 16, 1936, held at the Palmer House in Chicago, he took a list of actions already taken to comply with the recommendations from the two agencies.

1. The pathology department would handle all surgical specimens from the two Oxford hospitals for demonstration work with the sophomore class and for gross pathology and section tissue for microscopic study. In the next academic session, the department would handle all specimens from several other north Mississippi hospitals.

2. The pathology department would do autopsies free for any hospital in a 60–70 mile radius of Oxford.

3. Charity patients from the two Oxford hospitals would be assigned to sophomore students on definite schedules for taking histories, doing physical exams.

4. Hospitals in Houston, Tupelo and Grenada agreed to hold monthly or bimonthly all-day clinics for sophomore students.

5. Students would spend the last two weeks of the session attending clinics at Mississippi State Hospital at Whitfield, Charity Hospital in Jackson and the tuberculosis sanatorium in Magee.

With these changes in place, students would have ample opportunity for exposure to patients and autopsies in their first two years. Guyton also went armed with a resolution from the board of trustees that promised to seek a substantial increase in the medical school appropriation from the state legislature to comply with the recommendation for a bigger budget, increased faculty salaries, and more faculty.

The minutes of that meeting show that the school's status would remain unchanged (probation), but that the first-year students would be granted protection. Guyton's appeal paid off later.

In the spring of 1936, the legislature made a substantial appropriation for the school, and a freshman class of twenty enrolled. Sansing calls the growth and improvement in the school over the next two years "spectacular." By 1938, the medical school staff totaled thirty-three, a four-fold increase from the 1930–1931 session. With this infusion of money, the school completed the work on the building begun in 1929, added and equipped new laboratories, hired more faculty and more support staff, and increased the library holdings.

During the great rebuilding of the medical school, it was Dr. Peter Rowland, the medical school professor, so instrumental in the establishment of the school in 1903, who almost single-handedly amassed the resources to upgrade the school's library. The issue of the woefully inadequate medical library had been pivotal in the school's accreditation crisis. Rowland was almost a casualty of the Bilbo purge because of his age, but the board never got around to finding a replacement. In the second annual Billy S. Guyton History of Medicine Lecture at the Medical Center in 1995, Sansing said, "Rowland's methodology may have been unorthodox, but his acquisition skills were legendary." He traveled the state in a pickup truck, stopping in at physicians' offices and asking for donations for the library. In his honor the medical library is still called the Peter Rowland Medical Library. It was also Rowland who first expressed the dream, as early as 1905, of a teaching hospital and four-year school in Jackson.

Finally, after the better part of the decade, the AAMC removed the school from probationary status in November 1937, and the AMA reinstated the school as a fully accredited program of basic medical sciences in February 1938.

Dr. Billy Guyton was the man largely responsible for preserving and restoring the medical school. Dr. Julius Cruse, professor of pathology and Distinguished Professor of the History of Medicine at the Medical Center, said Guyton understood the importance of "that little two-year medical school." Had it failed during its time of crisis, the state would be light years away from having a full four-year program. "What we have today just would not exist were it not for Billy Guyton," Cruse said.

Cruse grew up knowing Guyton, or "Dr. Billy" as his friends had called him. Cruse's father was orphaned at the age of six when Cruse's grandparents died of typhoid fever. Billy Guyton saw to it that the children were placed in good homes. Cruse's father grew up in a physician's home in Ingomar, where the Guyton family owned a farm and where Billy Guyton had grown up. Dr. Billy stayed in touch first with Cruse's father and later with Cruse himself, taking an interest in both careers and lending a helping hand when he could. He often helped the precocious Cruse by writing letters of recommendation, including one for a Fulbright Scholarship, which Cruse won.

"I never knew anyone who commanded the respect that Dr. Billy did," Cruse said in a March 28, 2003, interview. "People who were his patients, those who knew him in the community, and other physicians all spoke of him with a kind of reverence not accorded anyone else."

A story related by Dr. Earl Kelly, the former executive director and treasurer of the Mississippi Baptist Convention Board, may explain why Guyton was held in such high esteem.

I grew up about thirty miles, as the crow flies, from Oxford, Mississippi, on a small red-hill farm near Ecru. Neither my mother nor father had the opportunity to attend school beyond the eighth grade. Even the type of education they received was in a one-teacher school where all grades were grouped together and sometimes the school year only lasted three months. As a small boy, I assumed my life would be similar to theirs—locked into a lifestyle that provided a very narrow horizon. Since my family had no influence or money, we were thought to be disenfranchised from higher education and could expect nothing beyond a rural parochial view of life.

My first remembrance of Dr. Billy Guyton was when I accompanied my mother to his offices, which were then over a store on the north side of the Courthouse Square in Oxford. Later, when I was about eleven years of age, in the early 1930s, my parents took me to Dr. Guyton for an eye examination. It turned out that I was suffering from astigmatism. The office outside his examining room was overflowing, yet he pulled a stool up in front of me and sat on it after he had completed the examination. He took time to visit with a country boy who was timid and who had lived on the brink of poverty all his life. He asked me about myself and my family. Then, looking me straight in the eyes, he said, "Son, a doctor can tell a whole lot more about a boy than the condition of his eyes when he looks deeply into that boy's eyes. I perceive that you have a great native intelligence, and, son, you can do anything in life that you make up your mind to do." I walked out of his office with a prescription to correct astigmatism, but more important, I was no longer destined to be a poor dirt farmer like generations before me had been. I was twelve feet tall and I knew I could be something more than I had ever dreamed before. Fifty-five years later I find myself still indebted to a great man for taking time to encourage "one of the least of these."

Guyton was born in Tippah County in 1884. His grandfather, Abraham Jenkins Guyton, settled in Tippah County in 1851. Just as many of Mississippi's pioneer families, the Guytons came from South Carolina. Family genealogical records show that two Guyton cousins, Nathaniel and Joseph, both French Huguenots, sailed from England and landed at Charleston, South Carolina, in 1750. Abraham Jenkins, the first to leave South Carolina for Mississippi, was the grandson of Joseph.

The future dean of the medical school was the oldest of eight children born to John Franklin Guyton, son of Abraham Jenkins Guyton. Billy Guyton's educational passage demonstrated a family tradition of helping younger siblings. He enrolled in the freshman class at Mississippi College in Clinton in 1901. He finished his freshman year in 1902, and his younger brother, John Franklin, entered MC as a freshman in the fall of 1902. Guyton himself was not among the MC sophomores returning in 1902. He was working in New Albany. In fact, he didn't start his second year until 1905. He apparently earned enough to pay his tuition and to help his siblings get their educational start. He graduated from MC in 1908. While there, he was active in all sorts of campus activities: business manager of the college yearbook, president of the Baptist Young People's Union, captain of the tennis team, and "critic" of the Philomatheon Society. Sansing found a mention of Guyton in the minutes of the literary society's meetings. "The minutes do not indicate what the duties of the critic might have been, but apparently Billy Guyton was busy demonstrating that if you can be responsible in little things, you can later be responsible in bigger things." Sansing says the minutes note, "One of the most pleasing features of the meeting was the report of the critic. For the first time in many months, the duty of the critic was performed as it should be."

Sansing said also that Billy Guyton taught in Dexter High School in Walthall County immediately after graduating from MC in order to amass the funds necessary to pay medical school tuition. No one is sure what changed his focus from banking to medicine, but his yearbook at Mississippi College called him "a banker of no little experience who intends to make that profession his life's work."

At the Ole Miss medical school, that was just five years old at the time Guyton entered, Guyton earned the MA in 1910 and the certificate in medicine in 1911.

He completed his medical education at the University of Virginia where his grades were high enough to earn him membership in Phi Beta Kappa.

Following his first year of internship at Martha Jefferson Sanatorium in Charlottesville, Virginia, he married Kate Smallwood of New Albany. Kate left for China as a missionary in 1908—the same year Billy graduated from MC—the youngest missionary ever sent by the Women's Board of the Southern Methodist Church. She spent five years in China teaching physics, chemistry, and mathematics. When Billy finished a year of internship at Orange Memorial Hospital in New Jersey, the couple returned to Ingomar, where Billy's parents lived, and seven miles from New Albany, the home of Kate's parents. The young physician practiced medicine as a "country doctor" in the small community of Ingomar—an experience that added to his understanding of the people of Mississippi and their needs. In 1915, he accepted an appointment to the faculty of the medical school at Ole Miss in Oxford where he also set up the Guyton Clinic. During summers, he took postgraduate training in ophthalmology at the University of Colorado. After several summer sessions, he received the Doctor of Ophthalmology. According to Sansing, Guyton was about to buy a home in Denver because the University of Colorado had offered him a post on its medical school faculty. But Billy's father, John Franklin Guyton "interceded and persuaded Billy to come back to Mississippi."

At the time of his appointment as dean in 1935, he had an active practice in eye, ear, nose and throat surgery in Oxford. He was a part-time teacher in the medical school from 1915 until 1926 in pathology and bacteriology, and from 1926 until 1935, in minor surgery and physical diagnosis. His experience as a teacher, as a physician with an active practice, as the loyal son of a pioneer farm family, his intellectual gifts and his personal integrity all combined to make him the perfect candidate to save the medical school. "He knew Mississippi and its people," Dr. Julius Cruse said. "He knew of the state's grinding poverty and the personal commitment of many people who had worked to keep the school open. He understood that if we couldn't preserve the two-year school, the state would lose the base on which to build what we have today."

Cruse points out that Guyton's job as dean was a far cry from that of his counterparts in other parts of the country where there was a long tradition of philanthropy for medical education. His success would depend on his ability to convince key people of the need for preserving the school, and he possessed the personal characteristics that made people believe him. But his job did not end when the crisis was over. Guyton, dean until 1944, presided over the most significant expansion program in the two-year medical school's history. The university named the medical building for Guyton in 1961 in appreciation for his vital role in saving and building the school.

After Guyton stepped down as dean in 1944, Chancellor John D. Williams appointed Guyton, Dr. David Wilson, and the new medical school dean Dr. David Pankratz as members of the first planning committee for a four-year school.

When the four-year school and teaching hospital opened in Jackson in 1955, Gutyon was dean emeritus. His influence proved far greater than his honorary title indicated. Were it not for him, the Medical Center's history would not have included the achievements of his son, Dr. Arthur Guyton, nor those of Dr. James D. Hardy. When Arthur Guyton contracted polio as a surgical resident at Massachusetts General Hospital, it was his father who brought Arthur back to Oxford and suggested that he stay close to home. He joined the faculty of the two-year school, now under the leadership of Dean Pankratz, and became chairman of physiology in 1948. Arthur Guyton came to Jackson in 1955 when the school moved and expanded, and it was in Jackson that his research would make him one of the world's leading physiologists, and his physiology textbook, which he started for students in Oxford, would become the best-selling medical textbook of all time.

James Hardy, one of the promising young academic physicians Pankratz recruited to be the first department chairs of the new four-year enterprise, brought international attention to the Medical Center for his historic transplants and for his leadership of nearly every national and international surgery society of note. He headed the team that did the first human lung transplant in 1963 and the team that transplanted a chimpanzee heart into a human in 1964. Hardy, already appointed by Dean Pankratz but still on faculty at the University of Tennessee in Memphis awaiting the completion of the medical school, was having second thoughts about making the move from Memphis to join the new Medical Center. Billy Guyton, now dean emeritus, got wind of Hardy's misgivings and asked Hardy if he could visit in Memphis to talk about it. The visit led to another by Chancellor Williams, and finally, the issues that had led to Hardy's equivocation were dispelled.

CHAPTER 3

Years of Transition

The accreditation crisis of the 1930s convinced university and medical school leaders that the two-year medical school as it existed in Oxford would never conform to the changing standards in medical education.

After World War II, the state faced an alarming shortage of physicians and hospital beds. In 1946, twenty-four counties had no hospital at all. In total, the state had only a third of the recommended four hospital beds for every thousand citizens. The situation fueled an ongoing discussion about developing a four-year medical school curriculum, and it had long been recognized that Oxford was not the best location for a teaching hospital and a four-year medical school. Rural as it was after the war, its sparse population could not assure the number of patients necessary for the clinical training of medical students. Fifty years later, an argument for having a teaching hospital in Oxford—with its unprecedented population boom—might be justified. But at the century's midpoint, Jackson—centrally located with the state's greatest population density—was the only logical location.

The idea of expanding the two-year curriculum began early in medical school history. Two years after it opened, Dr. Peter Rowland proposed to an audience of physicians at a Mississippi State Medical Association meeting in 1905 that a hospital be established in Jackson, operated by the Board of Trustees of Institutions of Higher Learning, that would provide the final two years of medical training to Mississippi students. Two years later, Chancellor Andrew A. Kincannon urged Rowland's proposal to the board, amending it only to specify that the state grant the university use of the old capitol building, which had fallen into disrepair. That request went nowhere, but in 1908, the charity hospital at Vicksburg was offered to Kincannon to be used as the medical school's teaching hospital. The "experiment" lasted only a year. By the time local physicians had undergone special refresher courses to prepare them to teach students and needed renovations on the building made, the hospital did not open for students until 1909. In 1910, the state legislature became embroiled in a dispute between state senators Theodore G. Bilbo and LeRoy Percy and failed to make a legislative appropriation for the Vicksburg hospital. The faculty had received no salaries for their services, so when the legislature adjourned without funding the project, they all resigned, and the hospital went back to the city of Vicksburg.

Proponents of the four-year school after World War II faced fierce opposition headed by the politically powerful Speaker of the House of Representatives Walter Sillers. In the struggle to manage Mississippi's health care crisis in the aftermath of the second world war, the Sillers faction believed the solution lay in more hospitals. Doctors, Sillers reasoned, would follow the hospitals. This faction won the first round. A bill establishing a four-year school passed the state legislature in 1946, but the powerful house speaker attached an amendment that postponed construction until a comprehensive hospital building program had gone into effect. It also gave the Board of Trustees of the Institutions of Higher Learning authority to name the location of the school and hospital.

The statewide hospital building program coincided with a national push for more and better hospital facilities that was being funded through the Hill-Burton Act of 1946. The state had to provide two dollars for every dollar the act provided, but the matching money could come from any source, including state appropriations. In five years, the state appropriated $30 million for hospital construction.

By 1950, supporters of the four-year school and teaching hospital had amassed such public support that the legislature passed the enabling law that created the University of Mississippi Medical Center in Jackson. The state furnished $4.5 million in appropriations, $1.5 million came from Hinds County, and Hill-Burton funding amounted to $3 million. The three key figures in the successful legislative fight were Dr. David S. Pankratz, named dean of the medical school in 1946; Dr. Henry Boswell, director of the Mississippi Sanatorium in Magee; and Dr. Felix Underwood, the state's chief health officer with the Department of Health.

The five years between legislation and occupancy of the new medical center were busy ones. A building had to be planned and built, clinical department heads recruited, the curriculum revamped to include two more years of instruction, the administrative structure worked out, and a hospital put into operation. University chancellor John Davis Williams created a committee charged with planning and developing the new university entity: Dr. David Wilson, Dean Pankratz, and Dean Emeritus Dr. Billy S. Guyton, who had played such a vital role in saving the accreditation of the two-year school.

On July 1, 1955, with the $9 million building almost finished, the Medical Center embarked on one prong of the three-fold mission assigned to it in 1950. The Medical Center's charge to render patient care had to begin on July 1 because the old charity hospital in Jackson was to close on June 30. Its teaching mission, with the exception of a few interns and residents, would have to wait until September when students began classes. The medical school and teaching hospital, with 491,498 square feet, was probably the biggest building in Mississippi. The original building was a T-shaped construction that had the medical school in its north wing and two hospital wings, east and west. Hardly anyone in 1955 could have imagined what would spring from that nucleus fifty years later.

During the building's planning stages, representatives of the architectural firm of Malveney, Naef and Overstreet had worked with Dean Pankratz and the medical school faculty in Oxford in the planning of the new school and hospital in Jackson. Dr. Thomas Brooks, then chairman of the Department of Preventive Medicine, recalled that he wanted student labs designed so that the instructor could see all the students from one vantage point. The architect came back with a cost estimate for the unobstructed view of students and told Brooks and the other department chairs that they could design the student labs as Brooks had specified, but that they could air condition the entire complex if they did not. Brooks said he and the others were aghast that air conditioning wasn't already included in the total cost. They had assumed a modern hospital and medical school would be air conditioned. Brooks recalled that it was Dr. Arthur Guyton, chairman of physiology and biophysics, who suggested that if money were the problem with getting air conditioning, they should cool areas as they could afford it, starting with animal labs, moving to the research labs, then the student labs and lecture rooms, and finally the offices of junior professors, senior professors, department heads and, if money were still available, the dean's office. Air conditioning was finally assured, and the original student labs, while not providing the exact vista Brooks wanted, at least were supported with small metal posts rather than large pillars.

The competition for space that has characterized life at the Medical Center for so long, actually began *in utero*. Another snafu in the design was apparent only after the building was finished—there was no space designated for labs and offices for faculty in the clinical departments—surgery, medicine, obstetrics and gynecology, and pediatrics. James D. Hardy, the newly appointed chairman of surgery, was teaching at the University of Tennessee while the Medical Center was under construction. During this time, he ran into Guyton and Dr. Louis Sulya, the chairman of biochemistry, at a meeting of the American Physiological Society in Chicago. As they met and talked about the new school under construction, Guyton and Sulya laughed when they asked Hardy if he had seen the space for his offices and labs in the architect's plan. In fact, there was none. Hardy attributed the omission to Pankratz' lack of experience in clinical medicine. According to Hardy, Pankratz never visualized a surgeon in any quarters except a patient's room or the surgical suite. But in 1955, many medical schools did not have full-time clinical faculty. Many schools still used town physicians who had practices with offices elsewhere, so if Pankratz overlooked the need for clinical office and lab space, he was not too far removed from what was widely practiced.

Hardy quickly negotiated with Sulya and Dr. William Hare, chairman of pathology, who both had offices and labs on the second floor of the north wing. Hardy ended up with adequate space, and once Pankratz was made aware of the problem, he told basic science departments to rearrange their space to make room for clinical personnel. The basic science departments who gave up their space to clinicians made it clear the space was only a loan. They wanted it back and eventually got it two decades later when the clinical sciences building opened in 1977. Appropriately enough, it was named the James D. Hardy Clinical Sciences Building.

On opening day in 1955, the brand-new state-of-the-art hospital had one medical unit, one surgical unit, one obstetrical unit, pediatrics, the newborn nursery, and ten operating rooms ready for patients.

Wilson, whose charge was to get the hospital up and running by July 1, occupied an office on the top floor of the Woolfolk Building in Jackson before the Medical Center was ready for occupancy. Wilson was assistant medical director of the Alameda County Institutions in Oakland, California, when Chancellor Williams asked him to help plan the new teaching hospital. A native of Yazoo City, Wilson had been assistant director of the Commission on Hospital Care in Chicago and had served as chief of the program planning section during the nation's massive hospital construction program made possible by the Hill-Burton Act funding. He was the first to serve as director of University Hospital. In 1969 he was appointed assistant director of the Medical Center in charge of special health planning, and in 1973 became the Medical Center's assistant vice chancellor. He was an Ole Miss graduate with an MD from Emory and the MPH from Yale. He had interned at Staten Island U.S. Public Health Service Hospital and served in the U.S. Public Health Service for eleven years. He served in the highest echelons of hospital administrators being at one time president of the American Hospital Association and the Mississippi Hospital Association. He was also a commissioner on the Joint Commission on the Accreditation of Hospitals. He died in 1988.

The first University Hospital was essentially his creation, although it has gone through many changes and developments in its response to rapid changes in health care. The original hospital, for instance, had not a single intensive care unit because the technology that would support continuous monitoring and the ability to rescue heart, lung, and kidney function did not exist in 1955. In 2004, the University Hospital is now four hospitals. One of those—the Wallace Conerly Critical Care Hospital—is nothing but intensive care units. The critical care hospital, completed in 2001, is a rarity among hospitals in the United States but is certain to become the standard in future hospital design. The stacked ICUs—one for medicine, cardiology (heart), surgery, and neurology-neurosurgery—are designed so that emergency services, diagnostic imaging, and surgery are just seconds away.

As part of his assignment to recruit key hospital personnel, early in 1954 Wilson hired Ruth Werner as the first director of nursing and Emelia Wellman as assistant director. Both stayed for some twenty years in their respective positions. Wilson and LaNelle Blackston (later Baxter), one of the first nursing supervisors, greeted the first patient, Diane Parker, a child from Duck Hill recovering from skin grafts. Blackston recalled the night before opening day when everyone was in a scramble with last-minute preparations for the big day. Wilson, she remembered, was busy late into the night of June 30 mopping up water from a leak in the ceiling in front of the elevator on the seventh floor. Maurine Twiss, who started work in August 1955 as the institution's first director of public information, covered the move for the *Jackson Daily News*, the local newspaper for which she was then features editor. "The law that established the Medical Center mandated that the hospital do a reasonable volume of free work . . . never less than one-half of the bed capacity for indigent patients. Another state statute forbade two charity hospitals in the same town, so charity had to close when University opened. It seems to me that is one reason that the University carried the charity connotation for so long," she said.

The development of intensive care at the Medical Center paralleled its development around the nation and the world. According to Stanley Joel Reiser in the 1992 summer issue of the *International Journal of Technology Assessment in Health Care,* three catastrophes brought about the concept of an ICU as a separate space within a hospital and manned by specially trained personnel—the Coconut Grove fire in Boston in 1942 that killed 491 and sent 39 survivors to Massachusetts General Hospital, the second world war, and the polio epidemic of the 1940s and 1950s, particularly in Copenhagen, Denmark, in 1952.

Some cases of polio paralyzed the muscles responsible for breathing, and so the major polio epidemics hurried the development of mechanical ventilation beginning with the ventilation tank or "iron lung" in 1929 and progressing to the manual operation of a ventilation bag attached to a cuffed endotracheal tube and a tracheostomy. By 1955, just as the Medical Center opened, the first electrically powered and cycled ventilators were developed. In 1956, Paul Zoll introduced the external defibrillator for the heart. In 1960

Belding Schribner introduced the teflon cannula and shunt that made kidney dialysis (developed by Willem Kolff in the 1940s) feasible for an extended period. These feats, which Reiser calls "technololgies of rescue," coupled with the ability to monitor physiologic functions from afar (developed during space exploration) and the computer's introduction to medicine in the 1960s that could both analyze the tremendous amounts of data from the monitors and alert the health care team when the data indicated an impending crisis, made ICUs possible.

The Medical Center's first ICU was a four-bed unit on 6West, set up some time in the 1960s when technology was readily available and a means of paying for it, through the newly funded federal programs of Medicare and Medicaid, made it feasible.

It moved to renovated space on the north wing of the third floor of the original building in 1971. It was here that the world of drugs and crime penetrated the Medical Center and made it reexamine its security for patients. On a hot August evening in 1981, two gunmen crashed open the doors of the unit and shot a patient in his bed while the medical and nursing staff—charged with the responsibility of healing him—watch horrified. The unit was already slated for change, scheduled to move into new quarters in the acute services wing when it was completed in 1982. This building housed the emergency department, new surgical suites, and a fully modern and fully secure ten-bed ICU.

Hardy, who had signed his contract in 1954 with the university to be chairman of the Department of Surgery, led the surgical team that performed the first surgical procedure in the new hospital, a herniorrhaphy. Hardy, who would gain international renown less than a decade later for his historic organ transplants, was assisted by seventeen other physicians who scrubbed in to be a part of a historic moment. From the roster of patients expected, Hardy said he and his team did not expect to have a surgical case on opening day, but a patient came to the emergency department with a groin hernia that had caused an intestinal obstruction. Hardy recalled that each surgeon placed or tied one stitch each so they could be a part of the history-making operation. The hospital opened without a single unit of blood in the blood bank, but by noon, the hospital staff had donated twelve of the twenty-three pints given that day.

Machiel Perkins, the first night supervisor in nursing service, recalled that on the night of July 1 she took the call from nursing service at Baptist Hospital just down the street that provided the names on that hospital's "addict list." "We were grateful, because I think all of them visited us (the emergency room) that night with their exotic ailments and requests for drugs to cure them."

The north wing was open to the surrounding woods for the first few weeks, and Perkins remembered seeing a large opossum on many nights when she had to go through the north wing to get to central supply.

As for their part in getting the hospital ready for patients, Wellman recalls that she and

Werner spent the months before the July 1955 opening visiting the nursing departments of several other academic medical centers to get ideas on the latest equipment, policies, and types of personnel the new hospital would require. When they weren't on the road, they were developing procedures to be used for the nursing care of patients and for personnel policies, setting salary scales, and ordering supplies and equipment for the departments. In March 1955, just four months before the opening, the two nursing directors moved to the seventh floor of the hospital from their temporary offices in the Woolfolk building.

Werner and Wellman also met with the chairman of the Department of Nursing Education on the Oxford campus, Christine Oglevee. All agreed that the department should wait a year before moving to Jackson. A year of operation would get all the kinks out of the system without the extra duty of teaching nursing students. Oglevee brought her students down in 1956, and the Department of Nursing became the School of Nursing in 1958 with Oglevee appointed as its first dean.

While Wilson had the hospital up and running with 121 active beds, the medical school in Oxford was packed and ready to move. At the final medical school faculty meeting in Oxford on July 18, 1955, Dr. James Rice, the chairman of pharmacology and chairman of the committee appointed to oversee the move to Jackson, reported that all supplies and equipment had been packed and were awaiting shipment.

Four days after students began classes, the medical school faculty assembled for the first time in Jackson at 11 A.M. on a Saturday, September 10. Pankratz presided and introduced all the heads of departments who, in turn, introduced members of their departments.

Moving the medical school was accomplished by will, muscle, and very little money. Irene Graham, hired in February 1955 as director of the Rowland Medical Library, was responsible for moving the library. Graham, who retired in 1986, actually moved the Rowland Medical Library twice. Once in 1955 and again in 1982 when it moved into the new Verner S. Holmes Learning Resource Center. The library as it exists today is largely the result of her vision. During the move to Jackson, she recalled that she requested boxes of a certain size for the move. "We needed boxes that would hold one shelf of books so that we could catalog them according to box number." In that way, library users could check out material and return it even during the move. "We never stopped operating," Graham said. Getting the boxes of a certain size proved more difficult. Finally, after much insistence, she got her boxes, she thinks, with financial help from Dr. Arthur Guyton and Dean Pankratz. "I found out that each department only had $200 for the move. That was why I kept seeing people move their departments in any old kind of van or pickup."

Graham also recalled her surprise at being able to move the library in time for the July opening. She knew the highest priority was getting the hospital ready; the library was way down the list of areas that had to open on July 1. She thought it would be several weeks or months after July before the library in Jackson would be ready. "I was coming to Jackson from Oxford nearly every weekend with the Chancellor and Dean Pankratz. At that time, Dr. Guyton [Arthur Guyton, chair of physiology] was working in Oxford while Dr. Hardy [James Hardy, chair of surgery] was busy with his scholarly pursuits in Jackson. They both wanted the library where they were." She explained that she could honestly report to both of them for most of the weeks between February and July, that there's no way the library could be moved any time soon "because it's just a hole in the ground filled with sand." She missed coming to Jackson one weekend because she was at a meeting. The next weekend she found the library nearly completed. "All of a sudden, it was nearly done." One of the workmen on the construction site asked her if she knew a man named Hardy. She said yes, she knew Dr. James Hardy. The workmen told her, "Well, he must have a lot of influence." Graham said Guyton lost little when the library moved. He had already finished with the indexes and abstracts which Hardy needed, so the indexes and abstracts were shipped first while Guyton used the journals and books in Oxford.

Guyton had his own move to make. He wanted to bring the machine shop from Oxford that he had inherited from a former professor at the two-year school. It consisted of some very heavy metal-working equipment that they had to move from the lab to a truck in Oxford and from the truck to the sixth floor of the north wing in Jackson. Dr. Elvin Smith, one of Guyton's earliest graduate students and now the executive vice president of Texas A & M University Health Science Center, tells the story about the move in his unpublished memoir of the early Guyton years. When Guyton and his helpers got to the elevator, they noted that the weight of their equipment exceeded the weight limit posted for the elevator. Guyton dispatched one of his assistants down the elevator shaft to measure the size of the elevator cables. As the assistant called out his measurements, Guyton did the calculations in his head and determined that the equipment could be safely lifted by elevator. "I'll take responsibility," he is reported to have said. The elevator did the job, and the machine shop still occupies the space where Guyton and his assistants moved it fifty years ago.

With the hospital open and running, the labs ready for research, and classrooms ready for teaching, the Medical Center began its first year. A 1955 press release mentioned the center's "pneumatic tubes rocketing from department to department in split-second communication, its television potential for surgery instruction, its atom-powered therapy machines." The administrative offices were temporarily located on the seventh floor while the north wing was being completed. Not everyone had telephones, and communication central was the cafeteria. Maurine Twiss recalled, "In those early months, internal communication was sketchy. We used to find people in the cafeteria. Everybody would go there for coffee, so we could usually find the people who didn't have telephones or secretaries." She also recalled the bond shared by those who were part of the beginning. "We all felt we were engaged in something which I believe, even then, we all realized was important. And it was exciting. Those of us who survived and the few who still survive have almost a blood kinship."

Twiss planned the formal public dedication of the Medical Center that took place on October 24, 1955, after the students, faculty, and staff had finally settled in. In the annual report for her department, she reported four thousand citizens toured the Medical Center that day, guided by medical students who were given an official holiday from classes. "I think every newspaper in the state used every scrap of information we sent them," she recalled. "Mississippians wanted to know everything about the Medical Center. They wanted to be proud of something the state did."

The scientific dedication followed the next year. Faculty members planned the program of scientific presentations, and Twiss planned the mechanics. The social hour before the formal dinner at the Heidelberg Hotel called for liquor, which was illegal in a dry state but readily available nonetheless. After a trip to one of the local bootleggers, she had enough libations on hand for the visiting scientists and physicians from other states for whom prohibition had ended several decades earlier. Almost everyone in Mississippi knew how to tuck a bottle under the arm inside a coat. But she had far more than what could be concealed under a coat. Transporting the contraband to the hotel from her car, she used an empty typewriter case and made more than one trip.

The Medical Center actively began its mission in providing education to physicians eleven months after the center opened. The first postgraduate seminar conducted by the School of Medicine in Jackson, June 7–8, 1956, was designed to give general practitioners a variety of topics they might find helpful in the daily practice of medicine. Dr. Louis F. Rittelmeyer chaired the postgraduate committee. Those attending heard presentations on leukemia, subacute bacterial endocarditis, a test for endocrine function, acute head injuries, acute abdominal injuries, the use of Roentgenograms, the diagnosis, cytology, biopsy, and treatment of carcinoma of the cervix, and childhood allergies and infectious diseases.

The first cancer seminar sponsored by the Medical Center was on December 4, 1958. The obstetrics and gynecology department played an active role in continuing education, offering "The First Symposium on Psychosomatic Obstetrics and Gynecology" in 1959. Dean Pankratz is quoted in the brochure announcing the course, "This symposium will cover practical methods of dealing with emotional complications in women with obstetrical and gynecological problems." Later that year, the department offered "Pregnancy, Childbirth and Breast-feeding," a course that featured a panel of faculty wives who discussed their methods of breast-feeding: Mrs. James D. Hardy with four children; Mrs. Warren Bell with two; Mrs. Herbert Langford with one child; and Mrs. Arthur C. Guyton with seven.

The faculty and staff assembled by Dean Pankratz and Chancellor Williams to run the fledgling Medical Center were young, energetic, and ambitious. Most were younger than thirty-five. Of the clinical chairmen, only Dr. Robert Snavely, chairman of the Department of Medicine, was older. He was forty in 1955. The youngest of the group was Dr. Sam B. Johnson, who at twenty-nine was appointed clinical professor and director of ophthalmology, then a division in the Department of Surgery. He was later appointed to the full-time faculty and became chairman of the Department of Ophthalmology. He was planning his retirement when he died in 2002. Most of the original chairs as well as the directors of key departments stayed until they retired, providing the Medical Center with a deep institutional memory and continuity.

At the administrative level were Dean Pankratz, who became director of the Medical Center in 1955, Wilson, the first hospital director, and Chancellor J. D. Williams, who took an active role in the running of the Medical Center, especially during the first few years. Williams set the tone for the relationship between the university chancellor and the director (later to be given the title of vice chancellor). Although he came to the Medical Center one day a week, a tradition picked up later by Chancellor Robert Khayat, he saw the Medical Center as a fully functioning semi-autonomous entity. Twiss remembered that Chancellor Williams often said, "The Medical Center is part of the university until it comes time to ask the legislature for money." He obviously thought the Medical Center could make a better case for its needs apart from the parent campus. Administrative organization was a particular strength of Williams, according to Twiss, and his guiding hand was absolutely necessary during the first few years in the Medical Center's life.

The department chairs who transferred from Oxford were Dr. Thomas Brooks, preventive medicine; Dr. Arthur Guyton, physiology and biophysics; Dr. William V. Hare, pathology; Dr. Ira D. Hogg, anatomy; Dr. Marcus E. Morrison, bacteriology (later microbiology); Dr. James Rice, pharmacology; Dr. L. L. Sulya, physiological chemistry (later biochemistry).

The new clinical department chairs in addition to Snavely were Dr. James D. Hardy, surgery; Dr. Michael Newton, obstetrics-gynecology; Dr. Blair Batson, pediatrics; and Dr. Robert D. Sloan, radiology. Dr. Warren Napier Bell was recruited as director of laboratories, which later became the Department of Clinical Laboratory Sciences. Hardy, Batson, Sloan, and Bell stayed at the Medical Center until they retired. Snavely died from cancer in 1964. Newton left the Medical Center in 1966 to become executive director of the American College of Obstetricians and Gynecologists.

Other key faculty members who came on board the first year were Dr. Fred Allison, chief of infectious diseases; Dr. Thomas M. (Peter) Blake, chief of cardiology; and Dr. Herbert Langford, chief of endocrinology, all in medicine; and Dr. Orlando Andy, the first neurosurgeon at the Medical Center. Andy later became chairman when neurosurgery became a department. He died in 1997. Dr. Glace Bittenbender was the first professor of anesthesiology, at that time still a division in the Department of Surgery. He died in 1957. Dr. Margaret Batson, first wife of Blair Batson, came with her husband in 1955 as assistant professor of pediatrics and director of the pediatric outpatient services. She died in 1998. The first chair of psychiatry wasn't filled until 1956 by Dr. Floy Jack (Flick) Moore. He was chair until 1968.

Key original support staff who spent their careers at the Medical Center were Irene Graham, director of the Rowland Medical Library; Maurine Twiss, director of public information; Frank Zimmerman, the center's comptroller; Lallah White, registrar; Fred McEwen, chief pharmacist, later director of the pharmacy; Clay Gordon, x-ray technician who later became director of the technician program; and Marie Louise Hoffman, director of social work. Fred White was the first director of the physical plant. The husband of registrar Lallah White, he died in 1957, succeeded by Ted Waldrom.

"All of us knew we were engaged in something important for the state," Twiss said. "It made us very close as a group."

As for the accomplishments of Arthur Guyton and James Hardy, it's rare for any institution to have two such giants on its faculty at the same time, and for this small new school in out-of-the-way Mississippi, it was just incredible luck and happy circumstance. When Dr. Robert Marston succeeded Pankratz in 1961 as dean and Medical Center director, he was keenly aware of the presence of the two men. He called Guyton a "giant" and Hardy "a rising star." And yet, there were still others in that original group who made notable contributions to medicine and science.

Herbert Langford helped to establish the Medical Center as a national player in clinical research. He was one of the key members of the landmark national study on high blood pressure funded by the National Institutes of Health, the Hypertension Detection and Followup Program. It was landmark because it proved, through following hundreds of patients all across the country, that treatment of what was then called "mild" hypertension could significantly reduce mortality from heart attack and stroke. He was instrumental in many such studies, helping formulate the design and execution of large epidemiological studies. Along the way, he was one of the first to note the difference in blood pressures among ethnic groups, and one of the first to establish the link between dietary salt intake and high blood pressure. Langford, a tidewater Virginian, urbane and handsome, often took his afternoon coffee in North Clinic (where physicians on faculty saw their private patients until the Pavilion was built) in the small paper cups used to collect urine samples. He called it the "perfect demitasse size." A vigorous athlete, he died suddenly in 1991 from a ruptured brain aneurysm.

Peter Blake, mentor to hundreds of students throughout the years, authored five editions of the medical textbook, *Practice of Electrocardiography*. He improved the care that physicians in Mississippi gave their patients by interpreting their EKGs by facsimile. When he wasn't teaching Introduction to Clinical Medicine, which influenced so many Mississippi physicians, he was at his desk, "reading Gs." Even after his formal "retirement," he worked as much as the retirement system would allow right up until cancer finally kept him away. Blake was also a photographer and documented the Medical Center's history pictorially for nearly five decades. He died in 2002.

Orlando Andy was the target of national negative media attention when he was accused of performing "psychosurgery" or brain surgery to control behavior. His pioneering procedures in the 1960s—deep brain stimulation—were too far ahead of their time to be appreciated. But he is now recognized by neurosurgeons as one who advanced the field of neurosurgery immeasurably. In 1977, Andy received the Pavlovian Society of America Award for the excellence of his body of research. Andy died in 1997.

Blair Batson, while never gaining a national reputation for research, was absolutely crucial to the advancement of pediatric care in the state. He was a tireless advocate for child health and welfare.

Tom Brooks, chairman of preventive medicine, was a noted authority on parasitic diseases and authored a key textbook on the subject, *Essentials of Medical Parisitology*.

Warren Bell came in 1954 to set up the clinical laboratory for the new hospital. The native of Victoria, Canada, was an unflagging supporter of the Medical Center and until his retirement in 1988 was responsible for the efficiency and quality of the burgeoning demand for laboratory services. He died in 1999.

Robert Sloan, chairman of radiology, was considered the "conscience" of the executive faculty. He has the distinction of heading up the first study on minority affairs at the Medical Center. Dean Robert Blount appointed him in 1971 because of Sloan's abiding interest in the recruitment and retention of minority students and faculty. Like Bell's department, radiology served the other clinical departments and their demand for x-rays and other diagnostic radiology services. He retired in 1992 and moved to New Mexico, but consented to come back for the Medical Center's fortieth anniversary celebration to speak. "What attracted us to this small school in a small southern rural state was simply the challenge of starting a new school. I would do the same thing again if I had the chance."

The man at the helm, David Schultz Pankratz, came to Oxford in 1939 as professor of anatomy. He was born on the Cheyenne-Arapaho Reservation in a half-sod house near Cordell, Oklahoma, the son of David M. Pankratz, a farmer, and Elizabeth Shultz Pankratz, a schoolteacher. They came from Kansas to settle the territory. He completed his elementary education in a one-room country school, attended high school for three years, then worked in the Kansas wheat fields for money to enroll in Bethel College. He transferred to Oklahoma University for his senior year and entered Kansas University School of Medicine in the fall of 1923. The following year, he taught biological sciences at Bethel.

He enrolled in summer courses at the University of Chicago in 1925 returning to Kansas as a graduate student and teacher of anatomy to earn his master's in 1927 and the PhD in 1929. He was a summer research fellow at Wistar Institute in 1928 and 1929 and became an assistant professor of anatomy at the University of Tennessee College of Medicine that fall. During the summer of every even year through 1936, he studied medicine at the University of Chicago, teaching at Tennessee during the academic year and alternate summers. He completed requirements for the MD at Chicago in 1938, at the end of a year's leave from Tennessee, and joined the faculty at Ole Miss one year later as professor of anatomy. He became assistant dean in 1945 and dean in 1946.

Pankratz, more than any other single individual, can be credited with the creation of the Medical Center. He pushed for its establishment, then directed the planning and construction. He was named first director of the University of Mississippi Medical Center, a title he held along with medical school dean, until he resigned in 1961 at age sixty-three, only to begin a psychiatry residency at the University of Tennessee. Pankratz always found it amusing that UT let him use his years as dean as substitute for an internship. In his meandering path from PhD to MD to dean, he had never done an internship—something Dr. James Hardy saw as a definite weakness in his training. Those who worked closely with him at the Medical Center remember him saying he couldn't wait to be a resident and complain to the dean at UT about a parking place. Evidently, the scramble for parking at the Medical Center began early. After completing his residency, Pankratz worked as a practicing psychiatrist in clinics in Tennessee and in Kansas until he retired to Oxford in 1972. He died there in 1980.

The qualifications he brought to his monumental task were a dogged persistence, his ability to form alliances with key people (such as Boswell and Underwood) who understood the importance of medical education, and his flair for identifying and recruiting the people who could move the Medical Center from a fledgling enterprise to a solid institution capable of turning out competent health professionals and meeting the changing needs in health care.

During the four years from his appointment as dean until the 1950 legislation enabling the establishment of the Medical Center, Dr. Thomas Brooks said Pankratz "wore out two Desotos" traveling the state generating support for the medical center. At the same time, he was scouting the nation in search of young professionals who would lead the clinical departments at the new medical school.

Dr. Blair Batson said the youth of the clinical team was no accident. He maintained that Pankratz deliberately selected young clinicians who were on track to be department chairs but weren't experienced enough to be offered a chair by more established schools. "I was told that Dr. Pankratz chose people who were not yet at the point of being recommended for chairmen, but were on the track to become department heads." According to Batson, Pankratz had seen other young four-year schools put major sums of money into the recruitment of well-known academic physicians as department chairs only to find that they picked up and left when they had a better offer or when things didn't suit them. "We didn't have the credentials to demand what he couldn't give us," Batson said.

When the medical school wing was named for Pankratz in 1993, Dr. Arthur Guyton shared his view of his former dean at the ceremony. "No one but Dr. Pankratz thought we could afford a medical school. He was the only one who had the real faith that we could have a four-year school. He said we could do it for approximately nothing, and we almost did."

There was very little money in those first few years, and Pankratz set a standard for making do that has characterized the fiscal operation of the Medical Center since. Sometimes, his frugality was extreme. Twiss recalled that Pankratz once made the arrangements for a trip to Chicago for him, Frank Zimmerman, the budget officer, and Dr. David Wilson, the hospital director. "They went up on the train, and Dave and Frank discovered that Dr. Pankratz had booked them all into one room of the YMCA."

Twiss shared her perceptions on the Pankratz administrative style in her taped conversation with the late Dr. Robert Currier in 2001. She observed Pankratz during the time some of the local physicians were angry at the Medical Center's private practice plan. The plan allowed the faculty physicians to earn as much as five thousand dollars from private patients in addition to their salary. Many saw it as a form of socialized medicine and subsidized salaries. "Dr. Pankratz would listen to them [the physicians] with the greatest of patience but he didn't ever change his mind. I always thought dealing with Dr. Panrkratz was sort of like pushing against a strong elastic barrier. He would give and give and give and then snap back to his original position." She considered this characteristic one of his strengths.

Twiss said that Pankratz possessed qualities that were vital in establishing the Medical Center. "In my opinion it [the Medical Center] might well not have been here if it weren't for this seemingly simple, seemingly self-effacing, seemingly unorganized man. All those adjectives probably apply and perhaps because of that, I think that the emotion, the feeling, that most of us who worked at the administrative level with him had towards him was a sort of affectionate exasperation or exasperated affection. A few of our colleagues, I think, mistook him for a limited, short-sighted fuddy duddy, who was comfortable only in a little bitty academic world. They may have seen him as a kind of bumbler, and it is true, he bumbled a lot. But if you watched him closely you found that he was bumbling to a plan, to a vision, and that he kept inching towards a goal.

"His paramount characteristic that was vital to the Medical Center was persistence. No flash, no dash, just persistence. You have only to look at his early years to see that this was a native characteristic. . . . I have one little memory of him that I think applies. One time he fished a tiny notebook out of his pocket, and he showed me where he had written down the title of a book he had just read. He flipped back, and there was page after page after page of book titles. He told me that when he was a boy in grade school he decided he was going to write down the title of every book he read as he read it and he had done it ever since. I think I smiled to myself when I saw it. It was an odd, kind of silly foible. But then I thought about it some more, and I realized that this was a strong clue to this man. He would set himself a course, and that's what he did. He just kept right on doing it."

When Robert Sloan spoke at the fortieth anniversary convocation, he reminisced about Pankratz. "I must confess," he said, "in the arrogance of my youth, I sometimes thought he was a senile old fuddy duddy. But he was a gentleman of the old school, and he came from simpler times. The more time I've had to reflect on what he accomplished and what he had to put up with has made me realize what a gift he was to this institution."

Sloan recounted a story about Pankratz that was perhaps indicative of the behavior that made his young faculty think of him as a "fuddy duddy."

"I was in his office to request some additional support for the radiology department. I was making a superb presentation, pounding my hand on the desk for emphasis and carefully outlining to the dean what I thought I needed. He turned his head from me and looked out the window. In the middle of my speech, the dean asked to no one that I could see, 'Why is that woman parking in a reserved space?' Needless to say, my presentation never quite recovered."

To Hardy, the young, ambitious surgery chair, the Pankratz method of administration was indirect and puzzling. Hardy was anything but indirect and hardly ever puzzling. Hardy's own writings reveal a planner, an organizer, a linear thinker who takes the most direct route from point A to point B. It is no wonder that Hardy found the meandering Pankratz puzzling.

Hardy was the first clinical chair appointed by Pankratz. As Hardy relates in his memoirs, his unconventional hiring was typical of the way Pankratz did things. Hardy had been at the University of Tennessee in Memphis since 1951. He visited Oxford several times to give seminars and to attend others, so the faculty knew him. Pankratz visited the medical school in Memphis frequently because he and the dean, Dr. Harwell Wilson, had been classmates at the University of Chicago. Pankratz invited Hardy to Oxford to discuss some of the clinical considerations that would be important in the four-year school. After four hours, in which Pankratz (according to Hardy) talked mostly about his experiences at the University of Chicago, Hardy left for Memphis puzzled by the invitation and the ensuing conversation. But in March of 1953, Hardy was surprised by a visit from Dr. Lowell T. Coggeshall, head of the medical school at the University of Chicago. Hardy did not know him, and Coggeshall did not introduce himself with his job title. He asked Hardy what he planned to do with his life. Hardy replied that he was going to "work like crazy," and if he wasn't a department chairman by the time he was forty-five, he was going into private practice. Coggeshall, in Memphis to address the graduating class the same day, pronounced him perhaps too ambitious. But apparently, Pankratz liked what he heard, and Hardy reports that one hour later, Pankratz arrived in his office to offer him the chair of surgery at the developing University of Mississippi Medical Center. Hardy said yes at once, but had several occasions to question his acceptance in the next few months.

In negotiating his contract (a contract in which Hardy required all members of the medical staff on his service to be board certified) he complained that Dean Pankratz would suggest one set of financial arrangements but then, "after another salvo from organized medicine in Jackson, would ask me if I would accept different arrangements."

When Hardy expressed his misgivings to David Wilson, Wilson gave Hardy his impressions of Pankratz. "I have come to know Dr. Pankratz well and to admire him. I have a great deal of respect for him and he has grown on me. At times he does appear to change. I think that is because he has the qualifications of certain strictly teacher types. I mean by that that sometimes he does not take some of the practical things in life too seriously. I believe, however, that you will find that he is loyal and will do everything he possibly can for your own good."

Hardy felt that the university had to enforce high standards from the very beginning if the medical school were ever to be a top-rung institution. He wanted all the staff surgeons to be board certified or board eligible. Most surgeons in the state were not board certified, and therefore would not be allowed to admit patients to University Hospital. It was a real sticking point with the community physicians, and Pankratz apparently was suggesting that a compromise might be made, but Hardy stood his ground. When Chancellor Williams asked Hardy for a final time, before he signed his contract, if he couldn't waive the board certification requirement for a few months, Hardy, who had been thinking for weeks how to convince the chancellor that it was necessary, asked Williams, "Who teaches PhD candidates?" To which Williams replied, "Other PhDs, of course." Hardy then asked, "How do you think a general practitioner can teach a fifth-year surgical resident to do major surgery? It is precisely the same situation as having simple graduates try to develop PhD candidates." Hardy said he had made his point with the chancellor and signed his contract that day.

Whatever differences Hardy and Pankratz had, they were not personal. Hardy viewed Pankratz as an honorable and devoted administrator and called him courageous for his practice of inviting heads of departments to have private interviews with Chancellor Williams. "It showed that he was not concerned about having different views expressed to his superior."

Dr. Thomas Brooks, the chairman of preventive medicine, related how he was hired by Pankratz in his taped interview in the Rowland Medical Library's Oral History Project. His hiring was as unconventional in its way as the hiring of Hardy. When Brooks was serving in the navy in 1946, his wife's mother sent them a newspaper clipping about efforts to establish a four-year school. "This appealed to me because I was from Starkville and my wife was from Yazoo City. I wrote Dr. Pankratz, and three days later I got a telegram from him that said welcome to the faculty. The letter said nothing about the effective date, nothing about rank or pay scale, just welcome." Brooks didn't meet Pankratz until March of 1947 when they had lunch together in downtown Jackson. Brooks says Representative Jamie Whitten was sitting across the aisle from them, and Pankratz said, "Jamie, I wish you'd get this man out of the navy. I need him." Brooks reported that two weeks later he was discharged.

Unconventional, unassuming, methodical while appearing haphazard, Pankratz nonetheless achieved what many had thought impossible in Mississippi. Yet, here they were in 1955, the first students who would graduate as the first MDs trained in Mississippi, the beginning of the promise that Pankratz had made the state if it would fund this unlikely venture. They reported for classes on September 6, the day after Labor Day. The total enrollment consisted of 135 medical students, two graduate students, fourteen interns, twelve residents, and three who audited classes.

The Class of 1957, the first class to graduate from the new four-year school, was made up of those students who had just finished two years in Oxford. It was a unique class in many ways. For one thing, they were almost as old as their teachers in the clinical departments. Dr. John Pearson, who retired from his practice in Hattiesburg, followed in the footsteps of his mentor and friend Dr. Thomas M. (Peter) Blake and specialized in the interpretation of EKGs. "They weren't much older than we were," he said of the faculty. Pearson said he didn't know whether it was their youthful enthusiasm as medical educators or the sense that they had to show success with their first graduating class, but the faculty "rode herd on us very tightly."

The clinical departments had to build intern and residency programs after they had faculty in place, so it took them a couple of years to be in a position to recruit housestaff. Because of the dearth of interns and residents, the members of the Class of 1957, who were seniors for two years for all practical purposes, did many tasks usually assigned to interns and residents further along in their medical training. The extra work made them clinically better prepared than many of their contemporaries. Jerald Hughes, who had a lifelong general practice in Bay Springs, Mississippi, recalled doing autopsies for ten dollars each at night and on weekends, work that would have been assigned to pathology residents or interns had there been enough eager postgraduates to do it. "I did more than one hundred autopsies in two years and learned a lot of medicine," Hughes recalled. Joe Walter Terry practiced general medicine in Canton until his retirement. "We actually did the lab work on some patients, something that would be done routinely by the lab now. We also did a lot of the work that interns and residents usually did," Terry said. As a result he felt confident because "I had confidence in my teachers." Fred Evans retired as a captain after a twenty-seven-year career in the U.S. Navy and then practiced ophthalmology in a group practice in Pensacola, Florida. "When I started my internship, I realized that I had much more clinical training than students from other schools." Stacy Davidson, an ophthalmologist in Cleveland, Mississippi, interned at Baylor, and it was there, in association with graduates of other medical schools, that he compared his training with that of others. "I had more clinical medicine and more exposure to patients than most of the others. I really began to appreciate the quality of my training."

They were also the class that saw Arthur Guyton's *Textbook of Medical Physiology* emerge from pages of single-spaced typed notes and hand-drawn illustrations to the first edition of what would become a legend in medical publishing, the largest-selling medical textbook of all time. Ralph Fortenberry, a family doctor in Prentiss, kept his notes Guyton made and handed out to students. "I learned more in that course than any other. He was a great teacher, and physiology is the basis for everything else you learn in medical school." Terry says he also kept his physiology notes. "I knew he was working on a book. I kept them as a memento."

Dr. Charles Allen, who by virtue of his place in the alphabet, was the very first graduate of the four-year school, is also a footnote in the history of Ole Miss for another reason: During his first year of medical school at Ole Miss, he was the first (and last) medical student ever elected Colonel Reb. He won in spite of a campaign that focused on the exemplary qualifications of his opponents.

"I tried to get my name off the ballot," Allen recalled. Brad Dye, former lieutenant governor, was the student body officer in charge of campus elections. "I went to Brad and told him I didn't deserve to be Colonel Reb, and that nobody would vote for me, and I didn't want my teachers to think I wasn't a serious student. He told me he agreed with me—I didn't deserve it and I wouldn't get more than a handful of votes, but it was too late to take my name off the ballot."

Allen's run for the title of Colonel Reb took on a life of its own. His classmate John Giordano recalled that someone got big flatbed trucks for night rides around the campus. Catfish supporters carrying torches would pull up to the dorms yelling, "Who you gonna vote for?" And the name of the reluctant candidate, known as Catfish since his college days, would thunder out of the dorm windows as voices boomed back, "Catfish!" Allen's insistence that he didn't deserve to be Colonel Reb stemmed from the fact that he'd done all his undergraduate work at Mississippi College and this was his first semester on the Ole Miss campus. He kept praising his opponent and telling voters how he'd "just hoboed up here from Mississippi College."

But the medical students who had decided to run their classmate were intent on having a little fun and managed to prove they could suspend serious study long enough to achieve some fairly impressive antics. An expert pilot—a member of the famous Key family in Meridian—loaded his plane with thousands of paper catfish, all with little parachutes attached. He dropped his payload over the grove where hundreds of students had gathered. "He swooped down just like he was making a bombing run, so smooth and easy, and the catfish were just everywhere."

Allen's photograph with Chancellor Williams and Dean Pankratz at the Medical Center's first commencement is part of the historical record of the Medical Center. Other members of that first class included William Arthur Brown Jr. of Natchez, Peter Louis DeRuiter of Edwards, John Campbell Gilliland of Jackson, John M. Giordano Jr. of Jackson, Warren W. Johnson of Ackerman, Hugh Richard Johnson Jr. of Columbia, Bobby Frank King of Oxford, Raymond Lewis of Eupora, Talbot Green McCormick Jr. of Forest (the summa cum laude graduate), Charles H. Martin of Kokomo, Henry Pipes Mills Jr. of Jackson, Charles Franklin Mitchell of Walnut Grove, John Miller Parker of Biloxi, Steven Lavelle Moore of Brandon, Nell J. Ryan of Vicksburg, Robert Lowery Thompson of Hattiesburg, and William Boyce White of Ripley. The nursing graduates listed in the 1957 commencement program were Laura Blair, Martha Small, and Mary Howard.

They and the classes that followed were proving to the state that their investment in home-grown medical education was paying off. In 1960, the Medical Center public information office reported that "In two years, 53 new Ole Miss doctors have started practice in Mississippi, accounting for all but seven of the 60 four-year graduates who've completed their training."

That first graduation was held at Murrah High school (which had also opened in 1955) in 1957. Maurine Twiss and registrar Lallah White, on instructions from Chancellor Williams, had made a trip to Oxford to observe the university's graduation so they could duplicate the ceremony in Jackson. At their meeting with the chancellor later to make sure they could handle all the arrangements, White, with a perfectly straight face, as Twiss recalled, told the chancellor they thought they could do it all with one exception. She didn't know where they were going to get a little yellow dog to trot across the platform in the middle of the ceremony. "Their exercises were in the Grove, and sure enough a little yellow dog had trotted across the platform with nobody paying much attention to it. I think I remember that because it showed the comfort level between the staff and J. D. Williams."

That first graduation in 1957 was as full of optimism and enthusiasm as the public dedication had been. The public was appreciative of this first class of MDs trained entirely at home. Three months earlier, Pankratz and his young team had achieved full accreditation by the Council of Medical Education and Hospitals of the American Medical Association and the Association of American Medical Colleges. The site team noted, however, that the Medical Center's current budget fell far short of its need, a financial state that would exist for several years thereafter.

While there was much about which to be optimistic in the first few years of its existence, the Medical Center also dealt with crises that threatened its future—conflicts with the town physicians, adverse public opinion relating to the transfer of a burned child, and financial uncertainty that all happened almost simultaneously.

For the first few years of Medical Center life, the conflict that was most consuming to administrators was the relationship with organized medicine in the community. There was a lingering resentment that not all physicians who practiced in the area could admit patients to the University Hospital. If their patients came to University Hospital, they had no say in their care. This was one of the sticking points with Dr. James Hardy, chairman of the Department of Surgery, who claims credit in his memoirs for persuading Chancellor Williams of the importance of having only board-certified physicians as members of the part-time faculty.

Another conflict, rooted more in economics that anything else, was the policy that allowed physicians on faculty to earn up to five thousand dollars a year in fees from private patients. Any amount above the five thousand dollars was to go back to the department.

According to Maurine Twiss, who was often on the front lines of the conflict because much of the acrimony was over physician "advertising," the conflict wasn't confined to Mississippi. "It was going on in nearly every state with a medical school because medical education was in a state of transition—from having part-time community physicians as faculty to having full-time salaried physicians as faculty."

The controversy was also a reflection of the national medical community's fear of "socialized medicine" in the wake of the growth of communism. In an exclamatory February 1956 article in *Medical Economics* called "Those Privately Practicing Professors!" Hugh C. Sherwood cites cases in California, Washington, Colorado, and Georgia in which the local medical societies were at odds with physicians in academic medicine because hospitals associated with medical schools in those states were treating private patients. His appraisal of Mississippi's conflict:

In 1950, construction of a new four-year medical school and teaching hospital was authorized. The State medical association promptly conferred with the school officials, urging employment of a "strict full time" faculty that would not practice privately. But the school (now open) has approved a "geographic full-time" plan which provides for private practice on campus and in the hospital.

It justifies the decision as a means of attracting high-grade teachers. And has ruled that no professor may earn more than $5,000 annually from private practice. Any excess is to go into a research fund.

Even so, Mississippi's physicians are up in arms. Dr. John P. Culpepper, their senior delegate to the AMA House of Delegates, introduced a resolution condemning "socialized and state subsidized medicine regardless of the form which it may assume." This triggered the AMA's current investigation of the problem.

The third aspect of the Medical Center's "town and gown" problem hinged on medical ethics and advertising rules created by the Central Medical Society (CMS) for its members. The membership of CMS, a component society of the Mississippi State Medical Association, was made up of physicians in the eight central Mississippi counties, including the three counties in the Jackson metropolitan area—Hinds, Madison, and Rankin. It was the way in which physicians on faculty at the Medical Center participated in organized medicine and their most important professional body of the time, the American Medical Association.

The fact that town-and-gown conflicts were not uncommon offered little comfort to those in the middle of the fray, or to physicians on the faculty who were threatened with censure by CMS. Censure, the least punishment the organization could dispense, was not taken lightly by Medical Center faculty. Michael Newton, ob-gyn chair, told James Hardy in a letter dated March 29, 1956, "A vote of censure on any member of the Medical Center Staff would set a very bad precedent. I believe that we should make every effort to prevent this."

It is difficult to understand, fifty years later—when hospitals advertise their special brand of healing in television commercials, and when physician practices "brand" themselves—how the listing of names in a local newspaper could spark such intense strife. Or perhaps it was just the proof to some in the medical community that the Medical Center was a company of elitists who would drive the practicing physician to the poor house when their paying patients leap-frogged over them to be treated at the Medical Center.

In truth, the opposition from organized medicine regarding Medical Center staffing policies, private practice rules, and physician "advertising" was generally from a small, but vocal, minority. When it came down to the censure of the dean, there weren't many in the Central Medical Society who had the stomach for it.

Maurine Twiss said that during her first week on the job she received what amounted to a public information policy written for the Medical Center by CMS members. The document, signed by Dr. Raymond Grenfell, then chairman of the CMS public relations committee, noted that it was permissible to use the University of Mississippi Medical Center name in newspaper articles about work in the basic sciences, and it enumerates the fields of physiology, pharmacology, bacteriology, chemistry, and anatomy. Not acceptable, however, was mentioning the Medical Center name in connection with any clinical work done at the center. Grants may be publicized, the document said, but the names of grant recipients must be omitted. No "staff man's" (physician on faculty) name could be mentioned in any case.

The society had its eye on the new Medical Center. Five years before the Medical Center opened, society representatives met with the Board of Trustees, Institutions of Higher Learning to discuss their concerns about the new medical venture in town. The rules, taken in part from the American Medical Association, but putting firmer strictures on the Medical Center, had obviously been made ready for the Medical Center opening.

In late October of 1955, Twiss met with Dr. H. C. Ricks, who was then president-elect of the Mississippi State Medical Association, of which CMS is a component society, to talk with him about the CMS guidelines. In a letter to Chancellor Williams, she reported an amicable meeting and found Ricks agreeable to compromise on the original CMS recommendations. "I am convinced that he [Dr. Ricks], personally, is sincerely eager to see the Center succeed," she wrote. Of particular interest to Twiss and other Medical Center administrators was the prohibition in the original recommendations that forbade the name of the institution in news reports of clinical work. To Twiss, these stories would be the very vehicle for allowing the public a glimpse at what the Medical Center could do and mean to the people of Mississippi. And, she reasoned, legislative support was often tied to public support. Neither she, Pankratz, nor any other physician on faculty ever really thought the physician's name should be used in connection with these stories. Although things would change dramatically in the next thirty years, at that time, naming physicians in news stories, except as grant recipients, was in blatant opposition to accepted medical ethics. But Pankratz did lobby for naming physicians if they were grant recipients, and he, like Twiss, wanted to tell Medical Center stories about clinical triumphs and let the world know where they happened.

These two points—naming grant recipients and reporting on clinical stories—were vital to the new Medical Center. Pankratz saw a public duty to report grants and clinical work because of the nature of the institution. Unlike a privately held hospital or school, the Medical Center belonged to the people of Mississippi. And many grants were often from nonprofit organizations that wanted their donors to know how their money was being spent.

Pankratz wrote to the public relations committee in October noting his disagreements. He offered to discuss the problem of mentioning names in connection with grants, but heard nothing. On January 3, 1956, with no advance notice or communication to the medical school, the CMS passed without dissenting votes a public relations policy prohibiting the naming of grant recipients. During the months between October and January, Pankratz had queried other medical schools with teaching hospitals. Ten schools responded; they all reported they released the names of the persons receiving the grant.

On January 19, 1956, the Board of Trustees, Institutions of Higher Learning, took up the issue, and affirmed the Medical Center–drafted policy for release of information to the lay media. The board agreed that using names in connection with grant announcements was not only in the public interest, insofar as many of the grants were paid for by funds made possible by taxpayers, but that it acted as an incentive to other investigators to secure more grant funding.

On February 3, Pankratz sent the Medical Center's public relations policy, as approved by the board, to the public relations committee of CMS. Hearing nothing for several weeks, the Medical Center public information office released a story about nine members of the faculty who received grants for research totaling $200,000—a fairly large sum in Mississippi in those days. Per published Medical Center policy, the release named the donor agency, the amount of the grant, a brief description of the purpose of the grant, the person receiving the grant, and his academic title. Grant recipients were Fred Allison, Warren Bell, Thomas Blake, Arthur Guyton, William V. Hare, James Hardy, James Hilton, T. D. Norman, and J. R. Snavely. Not surprisingly, the young Guyton received the lion's share of the $200,000. Grants for his work amounted to half the total received. The story appeared in the local papers on February 23. On March 12, the nine grant recipients all received letters from the censors committee of CMS calling their attention to what was considered an infraction of the local rules of ethics. They were threatened with censure.

Finally, after Pankratz' urging CMS to meet to discuss the matter, he read a statement at the April 3 meeting of CMS in which he assumed full responsibility for the grant story of February 23. He said that, until the matter was settled, the Medical Center would refrain from using the names of individuals who received grants in press releases. He did not make a promise that the names of grant recipients would never be released, as CMS interpreted his remarks three years later.

According to the April 1956 report to the board of trustees, in a summary of the actions taken by both sides, at that CMS meeting, it was moved that the dean be censored for his action. At some time before the meeting, the censors committee had decided to limit the censure attempt only to Pankratz. More than one hundred members voted against censoring Dr. Pankratz, and only a few voted to censor him—an indication that the animosity toward the Medical Center was not ubiquitous in the organization.

Apparently, however, the forces that fueled the first rift were simply simmering beneath the surface. The fire was still on. Three years later, CMS lobbed another missile to the dean and threatened him again with censure. The offending article (it appeared in the January 29, 1959, issue of the *Jackson Daily News*) was two columns wide, and three inches deep. The headline reads "Junior League Aids Hospital." It was actually released by the Junior League of Jackson in preparation for their annual Carnival Ball. In total, the article, which carries a one-column-wide photograph of Dean Pankratz, reads:

> "The Junior League orthopedic appliance program at the University Medical Center carries with it far-reaching benefits for the entire community," says Dr. D. S. Pankratz, director of the Medical Center. "The first purpose is, of course, to provide braces and crutches for patients who are unable to buy them. In so doing, the League helps the University fulfill its obligations to its patients and to its medical students. Additionally, these very orthopedic aids help speed the patient's return to normal living so that he need not become an economic burden on his family and the community."

The complainant said the article violated CMS rules about using the names of physicians in news articles. Maurine Twiss said her office had been issuing similar releases for three years (ever since the first censure threat) trying to abide by CMS rules. "We had to have an authority who would announce grants, especially if we couldn't use the names of the grant recipients." This was the Medical Center's compromise with CMS. When grants were received, Pankratz announced them, without giving names of the other individuals. When the Junior League called about a photo of Dr. Pankratz and a brief statement, Twiss foresaw nothing that would be noncompliant with CMS wishes.

Her office had, in the previous weeks, sent press releases to state media outlets about heart surgery performed at the Medical Center. One of them was about the first open-heart surgery in the state. Dr. James Hardy, the chief surgeon, was not mentioned in the press releases, per CMS rules. "They were accurate in every detail because I knew they'd come under close scrutiny," Twiss wrote Dr. Verner Holmes, then a member of the board of trustees. She believed the heart stories were the true source of the attack, but since they conformed to published standards, no one could complain about them.

When Dr. Pankratz was notified of the complaint, it was by phone call from the secretary of the medical society. A letter followed, which apologized for the rule infraction of not notifying in writing the person against whom the complaint was lodged, the name of the person who filed the complaint, and the reason. A month later, the secretary notified the dean that he had been instructed by the executive committee to advise the dean that the Medical Center practice of sending announcements to newspapers about new faculty members "is definitely against the spirit of the rules and regulations of the Society concerning publicity for new members. Since many of these new faculty members will be engaged to a limited extent in the private practice of medicine, the executive committee feels that they should be governed by the same rules of ethics in regard to publicity before they become members as they will be governed by after they become members."

This complaint, over which CMS had no authority because the new appointees weren't yet members of CMS, seemed to Twiss, however, to "change the complexion because it indicated a greater degree of active animosity than we'd thought present."

The board of trustees gave its full support to the Medical Center, and its members voiced the opinion that the Medical Center practice of announcing faculty was identical to practices of other institutions of higher learning in the state, and if it were not, would not be in compliance with standard practice for state universities.

This time, however, CMS put on a full-court press. Instead of bringing up the matter of censure again to its membership and risking defeat, the executive committee chose to turn the matter over to the Judicial Council of the Mississippi State Medical Association for a decision.

It is safe to assume that they knew the individuals who were members of the council. Why they thought they would have the support of one of them, Dr. Billy S.

Guyton, is a mystery. "Dr. Billy" was the man who had seen the medical school through the accreditation crisis of the 1930s and who had played such a pivotal role in the establishment of the Medical Center. We do not know what part he played in the final outcome. What we do know is that the well-reasoned and exquisitely balanced published decision is characteristic of everything else we know about Billy Guyton. The council set aside the charge against Dr. Pankratz and found that the CMS had not followed proper procedures in the matter. The council's interpretation of American Medical Association ethical guidelines were much more forgiving than those of CMS. The council quoted the AMA Judicial Council in 1952 as reporting: "In the ever-expanding field of medical public relations, no single phase has developed more than that which leads to the publication in national lay magazines and newspapers of stories of research or surgery. Such articles, where authoritatively prepared, usually tend to add to public confidence in the procedure described."

The ruling apparently took some of the air out of the vocal minority in CMS, but eruptions on a smaller scale continued for several years. The Medical Center public information office continued to abide by CMS rules for years afterward, and it wasn't until the late 1970s that physicians' names were used in news releases. The conflict with organized medicine was won by attrition. The opponents retired, faculty members (such as Dr. Carl Evers and Dr. Helen Turner) became leaders in the Central Medical Society and the State Medical Association, and medicine became such a growth industry that no one feared a loss of revenue from competition.

A letter to Twiss in 1959 from a local physician sums up the feelings of some of those in the medical community who opposed the policies of the Medical Center. He wrote:

"If we conservative, anti-socialists, anti-third party, anti-big government, pro-free enterprise, pro-individual initiative, privately practicing physicians who oppose subsidy and champion the philosophy of sink or swim on one's own merit could just get you to thinking straight and level, we'd have no bone of contention.

"The State Legislature passed an enabling act to build a four-year medical school to train doctors and to build a university hospital to take care of the full charity patients of the State of Mississippi. The excuse for research is an ivory-towered concoction. To have the State of Mississippi in competition with private enterprise individuals and its institutions competing with private institutions is morally and legally improper.

"It is unfair that the transient medical populace [the full-time faculty, presumably] at the University Medical Center should have so able an advertising agency such as yours to spread your false propaganda while the permanent practicing physicians of Jackson and Mississippi have neither the time, the funds, or the ability to waste on such projects."

He was under the impression, as were many in Mississippi, that the Medical Center was created for the purpose of treating charity patients. Twiss responded by pointing out that the enabling legislation says the Medical Center "shall be utilized to serve the people of Mississippi generally; shall be operated on the basis of charges for services rendered, but shall do a reasonable volume of free work . . ."

The controversy was not easy for the Medical Center, certainly not for Dr. Pankratz, who was temperamentally unsuited for such assaults. But at least, although the media was at the crux of the matter, the conflict wasn't aired in public.

Unfortunately, the same may not be said about the other major problem the Medical Center faced in its infancy. The incident that sparked the media attack before the Medical Center reached its first birthday (March of 1956) was the death of eighteen-month-old Rebecca Sue Little of Brandon. Its origins lay in the still fluid admissions policies of the teaching hospital, its financial crisis at the time, and the hostility of those in the community resentful of the new Medical Center.

Here is a synopsis of events taken from testimony in a legislative hearing and from newspaper accounts. The story ran with banner headlines from March 17 until March 27, with sporadic stories after that.

The child's father brought her to the university emergency room on March 16 on the advice of Brandon physician Dr. H. N. Holyfield, who admitted Mrs. Little to his hospital for treatment. Both Mrs. Little and Rebecca Sue were burned in a house fire.

The father, with a neighbor, drove to the ER. The resident on duty (full-time trauma teams on the premises were not standard in those days) gave her something for pain, wrapped her in a sterile sheet, and called for a bed. This is where there is a divergence of testimony. The father says he never said he wanted his daughter to be treated as a charity patient, saying later that he had two hundred dollars in cash in his pocket at the time. And yes, that would have been enough to cover several days in the hospital—even at the then outrageous cost of twenty-eight dollars per day. The staff in the ER testified they heard him and his neighbor say the family had no funds for care. Therefore, the resident thought Rebecca Sue was a service or charity patient. Finding that the service beds were all full, the resident told the father to take the baby to the charity hospital in Vicksburg. He told the father to keep her warm, and he said he would call the highway patrol for an escort. The highway patrol car never showed up, and the father, arriving in Vicksburg and asking directions, went to the wrong hospital (Mercy) where there were, of course, no arrangements made for transfer. Mercy called Charity, who was waiting for the child, and the father took her there. After she was admitted and treated, the surgeon told the father he thought she would recover, and that he could go home. Sadly, the little girl died several hours later.

David Wilson, the University Hospital director, said the resident acted according to standard practice at the time. He did not consider her an emergency case. Had he thought her life would have been endangered by the transfer, he would not have transferred her. The hospital had seen many similar cases in the time it had been operating and had transferred them without problems. There was no reason to believe that Rebecca Sue would not recover. Her burns were not extensive. It was later determined that she died, not from her burns, but from smoke inhalation. Wilson explained that this was rare, and that no known treatments were available had the resident predicted the problem.

One has to consider the predicament of the resident who ordered the transfer, who was never named. James Hardy, in his autobiography, *The Academic Surgeon*, says that earlier on the very same day the Littles came through the ER, he had told his chief resident to accept no more burn patients. "We had been getting chronic burn patients from all over the state. Such patients require prolonged hospitalization and this was intolerable with the limited beds available for maintaining approval of the several different specialty programs. Moreover, it impaired the quality of learning of the Medical students in our teaching 'laboratory.' Therefore, I had instructed my chief resident in general surgery to admit no more burn patients for the time being."

Later, during the ink deluge about the case, Governor J. P. Coleman took the blame for the child's death, saying he had ordered University Hospital ten days earlier to stop taking more service patients than the 175 beds allotted. At the time, the hospital was averaging about 196 charity patients a day, and hemorrhaging money as a result. "They [the hospital] are $250,000 in the red," he told a meeting of reporters. The hospital must now have an emergency appropriation to stay open, he said.

So the poor resident, with orders from his chief to take no more burn patients and with orders from administration (with orders from the governor) to take no more charity cases, he had no choice but to transfer, especially, if in his view, this was not a case of life or death.

The disgruntled physicians weighed in. It was Holyfield, the Little's doctor in Brandon, who called for an investigation while being quoted as saying there have been "a lot of complaints about operation of that hospital and it's about time the state or somebody looked into the situation."

And, although the Mississippi State Medical Association later said it had no official position in the matter, one of their members, who was quoted anonymously, said, "They [hospital officials] said the case of this child was not a good case for teaching purposes. But has the hospital turned down any cases from highway accidents? No. Because they are covered by insurance. Many of these cases are not suitable teaching cases either." And defending other local hospitals said, "These hospitals don't see anyone in a dying condition and turn them away. If the teaching hospital was so pushed for space it could have given the child emergency treatment and transferred it [to a Jackson hospital]."

The senate committee absolved the Medical Center on March 26, 1956, after hearing all the testimony. The committee determined that the hospital staff was at no fault in Rebecca Sue Little's death. The committee, in its opinion, showed a great understanding of the purpose of the Medical Center and great sympathy for its mission. Its major recommendation was that the hospital admissions policy be made clear to the public and to referring hospitals and physicians.

"This experience," Twiss wrote, "taught UMC administrators a bitter but valuable lesson about responsiveness to the public. Never again, in my tenure, did the hospital believe it could operate without scrutiny, nor did it ever again underestimate the importance of public opinion, the power of the press, or the role of professional public relations counsel."

What the committee understood, but which the public had trouble understanding, was the hospital's role in the state's charity care system. It was true that the hospital treated patients who had no means of paying for the care they received, as they were required to do by law. But it has always, from the beginning, treated more than was required. And yet, taking care of indigent patients is not and was not then its primary role.

University Hospital's heavy service caseload may have been unique to local hospitals not created as charity hospitals. However, it was by no means unique to the nation's teaching hospitals, which by 1950 were providing charity care estimated at $100,000,000—in the same era that youngsters could see a movie and buy popcorn and candy for twenty-five cents.

The nation's poor had always been the "teachers" of medical students in teaching hospitals. Teaching hospitals depended on the poor to provide students and residents with a variety of illness and injury to hone their clinical skills. In the days before third-party insurance was common, in the time before the creation of Medicare and Medicaid in 1964, teaching hospitals shared the burden of charity care with the nation's charity hospitals. The difference was that the sole responsibility of the charity hospitals was to care for indigent patients while the sole responsibility of teaching hospitals was the education of physicians. Charity patients were often accepted to teaching hospitals only after they met certain requirements that ensured they would be good teaching cases. Large and older teaching hospitals frequently saw more indigent patients than they were budgeted to treat, but they usually had endowments to cover such losses. Unfortunately, the young Medical Center had no wealthy bene-factors to create an endowment to serve as a rescue mechanism. And even though the state was generous with the little money it had, it was not enough to fund the whole cost. Teaching hospitals, especially in the 1940s and 1950s, began to depend on a certain percentage of paying patients to defray the cost of running the hospital. But in 1956, the physicians on faculty at the Medical Center weren't well known enough in the community to attract many private patients, and the town physicians didn't like it when they did.

The legislature did make an emergency appropriation after Coleman's appeal, and he directed the Budget Commission to give the Medical Center money when-ever Pankratz thought it was necessary. It wasn't a blank check, but it assured the Medical Center's survival in those first crucial years.

CHAPTER 4

A Giant Among Us

The Guyton era at the University of Mississippi and the University of Mississippi Medical Center ended abruptly with the sickening sound of metal crashing against metal on April 3, 2003. Dr. Arthur Guyton, professor emeritus of physiology and longtime chairman of the department, and his wife, Ruth, collided with another car on Highway 49 North while they were on their way to a restaurant in Pocahontas that served quail just the way they liked it. Guyton was pronounced dead at the scene. Ruth died one week later from her injuries.

The accident ended sixty-eight years of Guyton leadership that began when Guyton's father, Dr. Billy S. Guyton, became dean of the two-year medical school in Oxford in 1935. Billy Guyton reluctantly took the post of dean at a time when the school was faced with the very real possibility of losing its accreditation. His astute leadership assured its survival on the Oxford campus and its expansion when it moved to Jackson in 1955. At the time of his death in 1971 at the age of eighty-seven, his son had already made a name for himself in the scientific world and had played a major role in the development of the Medical Center.

During his career as chairman of the Department of Physiology and Biophysics, Arthur Guyton became one of the most highly regarded physiologists in the world and the author of the best-selling medical textbook of all time. He received virtually every honor the field of cardiovascular physiology can bestow, and scientists from around the world have made pilgrimages to his austere office on the sixth floor of the Medical Center for a chance to talk, and better, an opportunity to learn from the master. At latest count, twenty-seven of his former graduate students are the heads of physiology department the world over. At least six of the past presidents of the American Physiological Society are his former students. Even the phrase "Guytonian physiology," commonly used in most medical schools around the country, comes from the way Arthur Guyton taught physiology to an entire generation of scientists. He's the author of a staggering number of scientific papers (more than six hundred) and some forty books. What he accomplished in his career is nothing short of astonishing.

As important as his scientific contributions were, his importance in the growth and development of the Medical Center cannot be overemphasized. Dean Pankratz and Guyton's faculty colleagues at the two-year school admired and respected him and sought his opinion about the very fundamentals of building a new medical school and teaching hospital. After 1955, he was a vocal member of the long-range planning committee that helped assure the Medical Center's orderly growth. More than all that, however, Guyton just never did anything halfway. In the classroom, in the lab, in the conference room, Guyton was 100 percent there. He was the standard, and many who knew they could never measure up to his accomplishments have, nonetheless, been inspired by him to do great things. He gave the Medical Center—young, strapped for money, and located in a rural state commonly perceived as "unprogressive"—credibility. Surely, if Arthur Guyton worked here, it had to be an environment where any scientist could be productive.

He was born in 1919 in Oxford, four years after his father had accepted a part-time teaching post at the medical school and set up his eye, ear, nose, and throat practice.

His childhood was distinguishable only in its idyllic character. Oxford had a population of about two thousand during his boyhood, and the small town provided a safe haven for an adventurous spirit and curious mind. The scenes of his boyhood could have been painted by Norman Rockwell: Guyton speeding down Oxford streets on his bicycle, sitting backward; standing on the roof of a shed with an extra long piece of yo-yo string from daylight until dark, trying for a new world record; damming up a swimming hole; beating everyone at tennis on the clay courts at his house; paddling the canoe he built into the lake only to have it fall apart; and playing chess in the afternoon with William Faulkner.

In the 1930s of Arthur Guyton's boyhood, William Faulkner had already achieved a certain amount of literary recognition if not wide popular acclaim. *The Sound and the Fury* had been published in 1929, and *As I Lay Dying* came out in 1930. Faulkner was twenty-two years older than the young Guyton, but Guyton seemed to have earned Faulkner's respect. Medford Evans, writing about Oxford in the *Southwest Review* in the fall of 1929, described Faulkner as one "fellow townsmen make no pretense of being able to understand . . . He is one of the most talked about and most seldom talked to persons in the community." Guyton, it seems, was one of the few Oxford residents who did talk to Faulkner. Faulkner's stepson, Malcolm Franklin, even though a few years younger than Guyton, was among Arthur's group of friends. Guyton's friendship with Malcolm inevitably led to a meeting of Oxford's two geniuses. Guyton would go to the Faulkner home for birthday parties for Malcolm and his sister, and he remembers being "enthralled" with the stories the novelist told. Later, when Guyton and his friends wanted a swimming hole, they targeted the Faulkner property about half a mile away from Guyton's home as having the only appropriate gully for miles around. "All we had to do," Guyton recalled, "was build a small earthen dam across it to hold the rainwater." After gaining Faulkner's permission, a battalion of twelve- and thirteen-year-old boys spent most of one summer with buckets and shovels erecting the dam for a swimming hole they used for several years thereafter. During this time, while Faulkner was busy writing the Snopes trilogy, he wrote in the mornings and left his afternoons free. Chess was one of his favorite past-times but he apparently found himself without a chess partner and engaged the young Guyton. "He was very good at it, and always beat me," Guyton wrote. "But I learned more and more about it and eventually beat him," Guyton recalled.

The novelist would also take Malcolm and his friends (Guyton among them) to Memphis where he kept an airplane. Guyton recalls that they spent many hours flying over Memphis, and when not airborne, crawling around the airplanes. Guyton recalled that Faulkner's brother, Dean, also a pilot, was with them on many of these occasions. In 1935 Dean was killed in a crash during an air show and exhibition in Pontotoc.

As Guyton grew older, his passion for building grew. He wrote that as soon as construction began on Sardis Lake, he began building a sailboat. "It was the first body of water in north Mississippi that was really suitable for sailing." He built it in his parents' garage that faced a sidewalk on Lamar Street that was busy with foot traffic. As Faulkner passed the Guyton residence on his way home, he often stopped to chat with the boat builder. Even though it was Guyton, now eighteen or nineteen, who was building the boat, it was Faulkner who knew all about sailing . . . from books. He knew all the terms Guyton did not, and spent many hours in detailed discussions of sailing. When the boat was finished, Guyton invited Faulkner to sail with him on several occasions. "I don't think he had ever sailed before, but he enjoyed it immensely," Guyton wrote. Once again, the novelist regaled the other sailors with his talk about the art of sailing. No one on these excursions could have known that a short decade later, the boat would be of little value to its builder.

Guyton, after finishing first in his class at Ole Miss, went on to medical school at Harvard, service in the military, marriage and residency training in Boston where he contracted polio. When he came back to Oxford after his stay at Warm Springs, Georgia, Faulkner asked if he could buy the boat. Guyton asked his father and brothers if they wanted the boat, knowing that sailing was out the question for him now, but they did not, so he agreed to sell it to Faulkner for the cost of the materials.

Faulkner, however, gave him three times what he asked, saying it would cost him at least that much to have someone build a comparable boat.

Faulkner seemed to have recognized those qualities in his stepson's friend that made him a little more vivid than the other boys of his age. But then again, it took no special powers of perception to realize that he would achieve great things.

The children of Billy Guyton and Kate Smallwood Guyton—four in all—were very successful products of two devoted, intelligent parents. The lucky mingling of genes, a rich intellectual environment and loving supportive parents produced Jack Smallwood, oldest son, who followed his father's career path and became an ophthalmologist, ultimately the chairman of the Department of Ophthalmology at the Henry Ford Hospital in Detroit, Michigan; second son, William Franklin, an engineer who headed his own firm with offices in Austin and Houston, Texas; and Ruth Elizabeth, youngest child and only daughter, a mathematician who worked as a college teacher and statistician developing testing procedures for the Trident/Poseidon/Polaris submarine weapon systems. But it was Arthur, third son, who made the Guyton name known throughout the scientific world.

His was a particularly helpful and pragmatic intelligence as he applied it to tasks that made him an indispensable member of the Guyton household. His mother once recalled how, at the age of three, Arthur assigned himself the job of keeping up with the hats in the days when men wore hats and placed them on a hat rack when they entered the house. No one left without a hat, and it was always the right hat. By the time he was in high school, he did all the carpentry work around the house and his father's office and kept the home's oil furnace running. He had reassembled it after a repairman from Memphis had botched the job. He had watched an electrician wire a house, so thereafter, took care of all the wiring needs in his home.

One summer he found a college textbook on the mathematical analysis of electronic circuits, which he studied, and another on electronic physics, which he also studied. As Guyton himself wrote, "This training later turned out to be the basis of virtually all of the research work that we have done in our department during the past 40 years, because most of this has been based on a mathematical, physical understanding of the mechanics and control systems of the circulation. The mathematics of electronics and the electronic control systems utilize almost exactly the same principles that we later learned had also been discovered by the processes of evolution during the development of the human being."

He credited many of his teachers for inspiring him, not for what they taught him in the classroom, but for the opportunity they gave him for independent study.

Miss Clyde Lindsay, a math teacher, gave him a book on solid geometry, a subject not covered in class, and he learned it on his own. "She gave me a book, and I worked massive numbers of problems. Then she would check my work. The thing I learned mainly was how to learn mathematics entirely by myself without having a teacher other than someone simply to show me how to get started." Dr. Leon Wilbur, who went on to become chairman of the history department at the University of Southern Mississippi, taught an experimental class at University High School while working on his doctorate. The class was made up of top students in the eighth and ninth grades who did what Wilbur termed "contract" work. Apparently, Wilbur acted as a resource when the students needed help, but for the most part, left students on their own to finish assignments. "It was this responsibility that was exceedingly valuable to me as a student, and I believe also to all of the others in that class. Most important, it taught us to learn on our own, further reinforcing the lifetime desire to learn outside of the schoolroom."

Guyton also remembers R. C. Cook, who later became Dr. R. C. Cook, president of the University of Southern Mississippi, when he was principal of University High School. Unable to hire adequate teaching staff for the science program he wished for the school, Cook used teaching assistants from the teachers' training program at the university to help him teach physics. Absent from the classroom at least half the time because of his duties as principal, Cook managed to impart a valuable lesson nonetheless. "He arranged the material for us to study and the work for us to do, including making available to us appropriate material and laboratory equipment to do special projects on our own. We probably did not get as deep a course in physics as we would likely have gotten otherwise, but I do believe that we learned more physics that stuck with us throughout life than would have been possible had we had a proper physics teacher. In other words, the willingness of Mr. Cook to help us learn physics, not to teach us physics, taught all of those in that class an extra lesson over and above that one gets in a usual class."

Emily Whitehurst was the teacher who gave the ninth grader the lowest grade he had ever received in school—a C. Whitehurst, who later married Oxford attorney Phil Stone, close friend of Faulkner, taught English with a definite inclination toward literature. She told Guyton his C was because of his lackluster participation in classroom discussion, centered on novels and other literature. Stunned by the low grade, he asked her what he could do to bring up his grade. He thought literature was something people could read in their spare time. In the classroom, he wanted to learn the basics of writing, just as he had learned solid geometry on his own after his math teacher taught him the concepts. Whitehurst told him he might

A GIANT AMONG US

be able to bring up his grade if he wrote something and brought it to her. He did, and her estimation of him evidently soared. He ended the semester with an *A* average. At the University of Mississippi, he minored in English. He took the creative writing course for which he wrote a short story, and much to the chagrin of most of the English majors, the science superstar and electronics whiz kid won the university's short story prize for the year and an expense-paid trip to the Southern Literary Festival.

Perhaps his greatest teachers were his parents. He wrote that they would attempt to answer anything he asked, without bias or emotion. Even on questions about religion—and he apparently had many—his parents, devoted to the church, would try to separate for the young inquisitor what was belief, what was fact, what was supposition, and what they simply didn't know. His mother, the former missionary in China, was a devout Methodist but was knowledgeable about the world outside of Oxford, Mississippi, and told her young son that many of the world's religions had much to admire and respect. In other words, he was encouraged to do the one thing they knew he would do anyway, and that was to think it all through and come to his own conclusion. His conclusions seemed to have led him to a skepticism about religion, and that was perhaps the only area of disagreement between Arthur and Ruth. She, the daughter of the dean of the Yale Divinity School and chairman of the committee responsible for the Revised Standard Version of the Bible, grew up in the Lutheran church. Because there was no Lutheran church in Oxford, she went to the Methodist church with her mother-in-law and remained steadfastly Methodist all her life.

Apparently, Billy Guyton wasn't too alarmed when his young son expressed an interest in socialism—a word not uttered with anything but distaste in most households in Mississippi at that time. "In the idealism of my youth, I wondered whether some of the elements of socialism would not be very valuable. My father and I discussed the ascendancy of the American economy in the 1920s as well as what brought on the depression and what types of changes might be possible to prevent future depressions and whether some elements of socialism might be better than capitalism."

Kate was especially helpful to her youngest son when he undertook one of his many childhood projects. With her background in math and physics, she taught him the formula for calculating the amount of sheet fabric he would need to make parachutes for his toy soldiers. "I learned the formula years before I was taught it in school," he recalled. She also taught him the physics and chemistry of photography and film development when he expressed an interest in photography.

62

This then was the intellectual world of the young Arthur Guyton and the one that indelibly shaped his future. A gallery of supportive adults—parents, teachers, friends—surrounded him, giving him the tools of learning and the freedom to use them.

But he engaged the world with more than his intellect, great though it was. Guyton was a very physical person—athletic, competitive, aggressive. His first taste of mobility and freedom was the day he learned to ride his bicycle. From that day, he was free to explore the world of Oxford as he chose and to find the steepest hills that gave the biggest thrills. He swam; played tennis (and played to win); played football and crushed his nose; skied in the winter and water-skied in the summer. He sailed. All of that ended when he contracted polio. Paralysis is a horrible condition for everyone; for Arthur Guyton it must have been particularly cruel.

He wrote about the months leading up to his hospitalization after the infection made him sick and about the day in the hospital he knew he had polio.

He had married Ruth Weigle in June 1943, and they had the first of their ten children in April 1944. When David was born, Ruth was staying with her parents in New Haven, Connecticut, while Arthur was on the surgical staff of the U.S. Naval Medical Center in Bethesda. When he was transferred to the bacterial warfare center at Camp Detrick, Maryland, they moved to Braddock Heights, Maryland, where they lived for two years. He called it "one of the most delightful periods of our lives."

When the war was over, the young family moved back to the Boston area where Arthur was to continue his cardiac surgery residency at Massachusetts General Hospital that had been interrupted by military service. They were settling in for several years of additional surgical training and bought their first house in Wellesley. It was late spring of 1946, and their house was still under construction—scheduled to be completed in September. Ruth and David spent the summer with her parents at their summer cottage on Lake Sunapee in New Hampshire until the house was finished about the third week of September. For three weeks, the Guytons worked hard to get their house in order. He put a workshop in the basement, began to build furniture for the house, and acquired some machine-shop tools that he planned to use in making instruments for his research at Massachusetts General.

Three short weeks later, in October 1946, the infection that turned the family's life upside down overtook the young resident. He never lived in the Wellesley house again.

He reports that his first symptoms were "an uneasy" feeling and the "inability to sleep." Then he began having intense lower back pain. But the schedule of a resident was unforgiving. The work had to go on, patients had to be seen. So he was working hard every day and unable to sleep at night. Finally, after much pain, a high fever, sleep deprivation, and the stress of working while sick, Guyton went to the emergency room because he couldn't urinate.

The first diagnosis was even worse than polio. The doctors thought he had tuberculous meningitis, a uniformly fatal infection in the years before an appropriate antibiotic was developed. The physicians admitted him to the hospital for observation, and during the night, Guyton tried to reach for something on the table next to his bed with his left arm. The arm didn't move. He knew then it was polio, but writes that the realization "didn't disturb me as much as one might expect." He was grateful he didn't have tuberculous meningitis, and—with the pragmatism and analytical approach that characterized all the rest of his life—he lay in his hospital bed and calculated the odds. Two-thirds of all polio patients, he remembered, recover from most of the paralytic effects of the disease. Only one-third of polio patients has severe and lasting residual paralysis. "I was enough of an optimist to believe that I would be one of those who would not have a permanent state of paralysis."

It was not to be. As the weeks passed, it became obvious that his paralysis would be permanent, so he was transferred from Massachusetts General to Warm Springs, Georgia, where President Franklin Roosevelt first went in 1924 to gain strength after his bout with polio. In his seven months there, Guyton recovered some of his lost strength and mobility. He regained most of the use of his right arm. Part of his lower left arm and left leg showed improvement. He regained nearly full strength of his torso muscles. But with a right lower leg, left upper arm, and both shoulders totally paralyzed, he realized that a career in surgery was an impossibility. With one illness, a career and a whole roster of leisure activities were eliminated for Guyton. But resourceful as ever, he counted his strengths, and his interests, decided what was important and what was impossible, and planned the rest of his life.

The biggest factor in his plan was "Ruthie," the young Wellesley student Guyton married right after he graduated from Harvard Medical School after a six-month courtship. They were a perfect match. Intellectually, she was always at the top of her class. She, like her husband, came from a family steeped in the academic life. Her father, Dr. Luther Weigle, was the dean of the Yale Divinity School and a biblical scholar. Before Arthur started dating Ruth, he dated her friend, whom he seriously considered marrying. But after visiting in each other's homes, he decided he would not be happy with the "country club type of life" enjoyed by the girl's family. Ruth's family was very much like his own.

Arthur was smitten. All of his life, he talked about Ruth's cheerfulness, her vivacity and her ability to charm everyone. She matched his seriousness with laughter, and in his opinion, that made their family happy. In letters that he wrote to his father during their courtship—pragmatic as always—he also praised the shape of her pelvis as being right for childbearing. And in that, they were in total agreement. They both wanted lots of children.

Now that he knew he would be paralyzed with polio, he had to depend on Ruth for much more than her charm. Their second son, Robert, was born one month after Arthur came down with polio. Now she and her two boys were living in what Arthur called "rather squalid conditions" in Warm Springs during his time there so they could be together as a family. She assumed most of the lifting Arthur required and learned to drive long distances with Arthur and the two children. If they were going to pursue their dream of having many children, was Ruth up to meeting the physical challenges of child rearing alone?

She proved she was up to the task many times over. Their tenth child, Greg, was born in 1967, after they had been married twenty-four years and five days before her forty-fifth birthday.

During his stay at Warm Springs, he turned his affinity for mechanical solutions to the plight of those disabled by polio. In 1956, he won a Presidential Citation for the Development of Aids for Handicapped Persons. Based on what he had seen in Georgia, he designed an automatic locking and unlocking leg brace, a special hoist for moving patients from bed to chair or bath, and an improvement on the motorized wheelchair that used a joystick, still the most widely used chair of its kind.

Guyton got several job offers in Boston after doctors realized his paralysis would prevent a continuation of his surgical residency. The Department of Pediatrics offered him a pediatrics residency, and the chairman of the Department of Surgery offered him a job in his research laboratory. But the ice and snow of Massachusetts winters could be serious obstacles to someone on crutches, he reasoned. And besides, Oxford—the place of his very happy childhood—beckoned with its ice-free winters and loving parents who would be more than willing to help Ruth with the demands of motherhood.

So Guyton and his young family moved to Oxford in 1947, and he began teaching at the two-year medical school. He immediately set about establishing a research program. It was not as though research were a new idea to Guyton. If surgery was out, research was almost as good a way to spend a career. He already had a firm footing in research. By 1947, at age twenty-eight, he had already published in scientific journals several articles that were based on his research at Camp Detrick. During his second year of medical school at Harvard, the chairman of the Department of Biochemistry, Dr. Baird Hastings, gave the young student a lab next to his office. This was during World War II, and Hastings was away from school much of the time serving on national committees. Guyton, therefore, worked in the lab throughout medical school mostly uninstructed, trying out his own ideas and gaining invaluable experience. The biochemistry department had a machine shop and the first metal turning lathe he had ever used. At night, he designed several recording instruments that could be used on patients. He started building an electrical device that could measure blood pressure, a project that he revisited and completed when he was at Camp Detrick. He wrote, "One of the first commercial electronic pressure sensing apparatus for measuring arterial pressure in animals or humans came . . . as a direct descent of the apparatus that we had built during World War II."

At the bacteriological warfare research center at Camp Detrick, he also designed and built a particle counter to detect the presence of bacterial agents in the atmosphere. In many ways, this interlude in his surgical residency was highly profitable and personally enjoyable. He expressed some doubt about whether he would be able to contribute anything to the program at Camp Detrick, having little training in bacteriology. But his training in physical chemistry and his electronic wizardry quickly became invaluable to the work there. In fact, his ability to design and build research tools kept his services in demand throughout his tenure in the military, and building was always a passion of his.

During his surgical residency, before he went into the navy, he was doing research with Dr. Reginald Smithwick, who had devised a surgical technique for treating severely hypertensive patients, those whose blood pressure was so high it was life threatening.

He worked with Smithwick on sixty of these operations in which the Smithwick removed the nerve fibers that go to certain blood vessels. The procedure was based on the theory that high blood pressure was caused by excess nervous signals from the brain to the heart and peripheral blood vessels. Guyton had relentlessly pursued the origins of high blood pressure since medical school, and this extracurricular research with Smithwick dovetailed with his quest. Unfortunately, though the immediate results confirmed the "neruogenic" theory of the control of blood pressure, the long-term results did not. After months or sometimes a year, the blood pressure in the surgical patients went back up. The operations extended their lives because they no longer got the exacerbations of blood pressure when they exercised or got excited, but the surgery had no effect at all on long-term blood pressure.

Although long-term results were disappointing, Guyton was still convinced that the nervous system controlled blood pressure in some way, and when he was ready to start his own research program in Oxford, he started with experiments designed to prove this hypothesis. All of them failed. They showed that the nervous system did have some influence on the control of blood pressure in the short term, but none at all on the long-term blood pressure. And that really was the elusive answer Guyton sought—the key to why some people have sustained, elevated blood pressure most of their lives with no apparent causative factor.

It was then that Guyton realized he had to get back to the basics to learn what controlled circulation and blood pressure. He successfully worked out most of the basics during the next ten years—the decade that it took him to get back to his original question of what causes high blood pressure.

In addition to his research, there was also a department to run. A year after going back to Oxford to teach in the medical school, the chairman of the physiology department left, and Guyton applied for the position. He said that Dean David Pankratz had many misgivings about appointing him because he thought Guyton's physical condition could not withstand the rigors of running a department. Happily, and to no surprise to Guyton himself, he had no trouble at all. "There were always people in the department who could do the physical tasks I couldn't do," he wrote. He became chairman in 1948, and that was his job for forty-one years until his retirement in 1989.

Dr. Julius Cruse, professor of pathology at the Medical Center and a long-time family friend of the Guytons, tells the story about Arthur's first year back at Oxford as it was told to him by Dr. Nicholas DiLuzio, who was professor of physiology at the University of Tennessee in Memphis when Cruse was a student there. According to DiLuzio, when his father first brought Arthur back to Oxford, there was no opening in physiology, so Dr. Billy Guyton asked his friend, Dr. O. W. Hyman, the dean of the medical school at the University of Tennessee in Memphis, about hiring Arthur on a temporary basis until something became available in Oxford. Dr. Tommy Nash, then dean of the Graduate School at UT Memphis, told DiLuzio that he would like to give Arthur a position in physiology, but then said, "he's not a physiologist." It was true that Arthur had no formal training in physiology beyond that taught to every medical student, but Nash's words would come back to haunt him. Instead, he gave Arthur a temporary teaching position in pharmacology until a place opened up for him in Oxford.

He played a remarkably large role for a department chair in the creation and establishment of the four-year medical school in Jackson. For one so young (in 1948 he was only twenty-nine), he also had a variety of experiences in both research and clinical medicine that proved immensely helpful in the planning of the Medical

Center. He was also the recipient of the university's first grant for research. Pankratz had money in the budget for Guyton to hire another teacher for the physiology department, but Guyton asked and got permission to use the personnel allocation for research equipment instead. With a well-equipped laboratory and a constant flow of well-thought-out research problems to solve, getting grant money was no problem for him. His success was a catalyst that encouraged the school to view solid research as an attainable goal, and led to a flurry of grant requests and acquisitions from other faculty members.

After 1950, when planning for the four-year school occupied much discussion in the executive faculty meetings, Guyton was the one who came up with the resolution calling for "a logical and scientific pattern" in the planning. He proposed that before real planning could take place, they would need to establish the number of people who would work in each department, the number of hours each member of the faculty would teach, the amount of laboratory work that would be done by each division, and finally what relationship would exist between the director of the hospital and the director of the Medical Center. He proposed that statistical information on the allocation of space in other medical schools be used to determine allocation in the new Medical Center. He also proposed that the faculty must approve the creation and organization of new departments "because the number of departments and the distribution of subject matter to be taught in each department greatly affect other departments."

As to the relationship between hospital director and Medical Center director, he suggested that the hospital director "be totally responsible" to the dean and faculty. His resolution passed without dissent in 1951. More than a half century later, the hospital director still answers to the vice chancellor of the Medical Center, an administrative structure that hasn't always pleased hospital directors but has made the Medical Center a cohesive unit instead of competing entities.

The July 11, 1951, minutes of the executive faculty show that the faculty was in "complete agreement" on the order in which the new Medical Center would be air conditioned. If money was too short for full air conditioning, the order of priority would be animal rooms, classrooms, library, and finally, administrative offices. According to Dr. Thomas Brooks, chairman of the Department of Preventive Medicine at the two-year school, it was Guyton who came up with the order, demonstrating what he perceived as essentials.

Although he had already written many articles that had been published in scientific journals, it was during his years in Oxford that he began his *Textbook of Medical Physiology*, the first edition of which came out in 1956, a year after the Medical

Center opened. The final edition with Guyton as author, number ten, came out in 2000. Guyton's successor as department chair, Dr. John Hall, began working with Guyton on the ninth edition. Until the ninth edition, the book was a rarity in medical publishing having only one writer. It is, by far, the best-selling physiology textbook ever published, and possibly the best-selling medical textbook of any kind. Hall estimated that each edition sells from 140,000 to 150,000 copies.

The book began as notes for his students. In the late 1940s and early 1950s, medical education was in overdrive trying to accommodate veterans who had postponed their education to serve in the military. The university's medical school was admitting two classes a year—one in July and one in January. Guyton, the only teacher in the physiology department in Oxford for the first two or three years he was there, was teaching all of physiology not just once but twice. As Guyton recalled, they covered vast amounts of information very quickly. "I changed textbooks with almost every class, hoping to find one book that the students would indeed study with pleasure and with depth of understanding." Guyton painted a picture of his classroom that was pretty typical—he, drawing diagrams to explain functions in physiology and explaining both broad concepts and details of function, the students with heads down, pens busily transcribing the lecture each in his own individual note-taking style. "If the tests asked details about specific items that had been listed one-by-one in the lectures, the students did very well. Yet any time a question was beyond that level, especially about some basic physiological principle discussed in detail in their text . . . their knowledge of physiology suddenly failed entirely."

He bargained with the students, telling them if they would focus their attention on him while he lectured, he would give them notes to study. After the lecture, he went back to his office and dictated the important points of the lecture. His secretary typed and duplicated the notes, and Guyton had them ready for the 10 A.M. class the next day. The students responded well to the notes and did very well on exams that were based on the notes. However, Guyton said they never looked at the textbook he had ordered for the class because they didn't want to be "confused" by it. Guyton was fearful that the amount of physiology they were learning just from the notes would not sustain them through the rest of medical school and the practice of medicine. So he expanded his notes to concepts and details not covered in the lecture, incorporating diagrams and charts and anatomical drawings. According to Guyton, "this worked beautifully . . . but it meant, however, that the students no longer looked at a commercial textbook of physiology and that they were not familiar even with the physiology textbooks that were available. In other words, the students left our school trained in the field of medical physiology as conceived and presented at the University of Mississippi School of Medicine. They were not trained in the depths of the worldwide scheme of physiology."

For several years, Guyton's "Physiology Syllabus" served as the only textbook students would read in their physiology course. It proved adequate.

At some point in the early 1950s, a representative from W. B. Saunders publishing company visited the physiology chairman and tried to sell Guyton one of his company's books. The representative, instead, discovered Guyton's syllabus, and asked if he could send it to Saunders's medical editor, John Dusseau. Two weeks later, Dusseau called Guyton to see if the author would be interested in revising the syllabus into a textbook. Guyton said he quickly calculated the number of hours he would have to spend on the book to get an estimate of how much additional income he could expect. "On an hourly basis, I would make an extra amount of money approximately equal to what a good ditch digger might make." He wasn't then, and never was, motivated by money, but he later remarked, half jokingly, that he kept writing the book, edition after edition, because he had to finance the medical education of his ten children.

The book's immense popularity around the world is due largely to the author's intention to instruct. It is written for students, not for other physiologists. Although many times more voluminous than the notes from which it sprang, the book's tone in the tenth edition was the same as it was in the notes. "It always maintains the tone of a teacher talking to students," said William R. Schmitt, editor-in-chief of medical textbooks at Harcourt Health Services at the time of the publication of the tenth edition in 2000. Harcourt was Saunders's successor in publishing the book. Translated into twelve foreign languages, the book is known throughout the world where students study medicine. In 1996, Guyton received the nation's top award in medical education, given for his contributions to medical education through the continuous authorship of the *Textbook of Medical Physiology*. The printed program for the awards ceremony at a meeting of the Association of American Medical Colleges described the time Guyton was in Mexico and "was honored with a sign of devotion reserved usually for musical performers and movie stars, and certainly rarely bestowed upon medical educators. When leaving a Mexico City medical school, a crowd of students gathered to chant his name, repeatedly calling out, 'Guyton, Guyton, Guyton.'"

The continuous work on the book meant that Guyton's workday rarely ended before 10 P.M. Until his retirement, he did all his work on the book at home, saving the days for the administrative tasks and research. He dictated his writing and revi-

sions then gave the tapes to his secretary in the morning. One of his longtime secretaries, Billie Howard, said she often heard the sounds of the children playing in
the background.

Schmitt, Harcourt's medical editor, said he learned he never had to worry about
Guyton missing a deadline. "Sometimes I will panic," he said at the publication of
the tenth edition, "because I remember that it's been a while since the last edition,
and I'll call Dr. Guyton to tell him it's about time for another edition. He will have
been making revisions since the last edition, and he always says he can send it when-
ever we want it."

Much of what is in the textbook is original with Guyton and his colleagues, the
results of work done in the labs on the sixth floor of the Medical Center, where
the physiology department has been since 1955. Other material in the book is
from research done in the other labs around the country and the world that was
spawned in the UMC physiology department. His early graduate students recall
Saturday morning sessions during which Guyton insisted that every student
present at least one new idea for a research project, and Guyton, too, presented
his ideas. One of those students was Dr. Aubrey Taylor, the distinguished professor of physiology at the University of South Alabama who retired as chairman of
the department there. The author of more than 450 papers and five books, Taylor
himself is a well-known physiologist. According to Taylor, Guyton had a way of
recognizing an idea for research that could make a scientist productive for his or
her entire career, then match the idea to the qualities and attributes of the student. In 1989, Taylor wrote, "I am still working in an area into which Dr. Guyton
placed me almost 30 years ago." Considering the number of graduate students
who came through the department and Guyton's influence on them, even in death,
his fertile brain is indirectly responsible for new knowledge about circulatory
function.

Dr. Elvin Smith, the executive vice president of Texas A & M University Health
Science Center and former professor in the department of medical physiology at
Texas A & M, was also one of those early graduate students. He recalled the Saturday morning sessions as a fountainhead of ideas for research. He remembers Guyton
trying to persuade the students to adopt his habit of writing down ideas for research when they come to you, even in the middle of the night. Guyton recorded all
of his own ideas on a piece of paper he kept at his bedside, and then moved them to
a file in his desk. Smith says many students went to Guyton's office to discuss an
idea they had, only to find that the chairman himself had given the problem some
thought and kept it in his special file until it became useful. "At this very moment,

there are enough research ideas, located in that file in Guyton's office, to keep many researchers busy, and remarkably productive, for the rest of their lives."

The book was a constant in his life after 1956. He wrote, edited, revised, and read widely in fields outside cardiovascular physiology up until his death. Another constant was his quest, begun in medical school, for the answer to the question of what causes high blood pressure.

In the years before 1955, in discussions with the faculty and the dean about how the new Medical Center should be configured, Guyton—with his dual interest in clinical medicine and basic research—always stressed the importance of a close relationship between the basic sciences (physiologists, biochemists, anatomists, microbiologists) and the clinicians who saw the sciences at work in the diseases and conditions of their patients. His primary research concern was hypertension (high blood pressure). He wrote that when he was in medical school, his teachers could describe what high blood pressure was, but no one could tell him the cause. After the surgical procedures he performed with Dr. Reginald Smithwick failed to produce an answer to the long-term control of blood pressure, he said he realized that it wasn't a failure of the research so much as simply a lack of knowledge in general about circulatory function. If he were ever to find the cause of high blood pressure, he would have to answer far more basic questions about the cardiovascular system.

He said he was "lucky" to start out in cardiovascular physiology when he did because "it was a mess," he recalled. "The two big names in the field both believed that the heart controlled cardiac output—the amount of blood pumped by the heart. But they disliked each other and fought constantly about just how the heart did it."

In the decade of the 1950s, there was simply no solid evidence to support a unified theory of circulation. In his starting-over period, he first tackled the question of cardiac output. "There was overall confusion of what constitutes the regulation of venous return." In lay terms, what determines how much blood the veins send back to the heart to be pumped out again through the arteries?

When Guyton began his studies on venous return, the prevailing theory was that the amount of blood pumped by the heart (cardiac output) was determined by the pumping capacity of the heart itself—or by some mechanism of the nervous system that controlled the heart and its pumping ability. In a series of experiments in the 1950s, he was to develop the theory that the heart would pump only what was delivered to it through the veins. In experiments, he replaced the heart with an external pump, and "every factor that we could think of that affected venous return was studied ... It quickly became apparent (from analyzing the data) that as long as the heart functions normally, most of the minute-by-minute, hour-by-hour, and even day-by-day control of cardiac output is vested in the peripheral tissues, not in the heart." When body tissues need extra blood flow to carry the required oxygen and other nutrients, the blood vessels in those tissues expand, or dilate, to allow increased flow. Therefore, the blood returning to the heart increases, and the heart, in turn, pumps the blood back around the circuit again.

Guyton describes his foray into cardiac output as a "valuable detour," one that had "begun to emphasize the importance of the circulation as a servant of the body rather than as master of the body." And it significantly advanced the understanding of circulatory function. The full explanation of this work is in his book, *Circulatory Physiology: Cardiac Output and Its Regulation*, the first edition published by W. B. Saunders in 1963. Other physiologists gradually gave up the notion of the heart's control of cardiac output, and now his explanation is in most textbooks, even in those not authored by him.

Since so much of Guyton's work concerned body fluids, he had to work out a description of the interstitial fluid. Approximately one-sixth of the body consists of infinitesimally small spaces between cells, which collectively are called the interstitium. The fluid in these spaces is the interstitial fluid. When the volume of this fluid increases, edema and swelling occur. This was one of the problems Guyton worked on as a medical student in Dr. Baird Hastings's lab. He came to believe, even then, that contrary to what he was taught, the normal pressure in interstitial fluid was subatmospheric or negative, that the lymphatic system, under normal conditions, was constantly sucking the fluid from between the cells into the lymphatic vessels. In his words, "We aren't a blown-up balloon, but a sucked-dry balloon." His own logic led him to this conclusion from evidence he saw as a surgical resident. For instance, when skin grafts were placed in the eye sockets of patients whose eyes had been removed, fluid collected underneath the skin, but was eventually absorbed and the skin pulled even farther back into the eye socket. "This could not have happened without a strong negative pressure within that fluid."

But proof of his logic had to wait twenty years before he could demonstrate it to a scientific community virtually incapable of accepting it. He first had to design a device whereby the tiny space could be entered and the pressure measured, finally arriving at a perforated plastic capsule surgically implanted. The capsule created an artificial space within the interstitium, but a space that had all the characteristics of the natural. Just as he had predicted, the pressure was negative. That finding led to many others that clarified the mechanisms of edema and congestive heart failure, and it opened up many other areas of study that were now possible because of this new knowledge. His findings led to much spirited debate at national meetings where Guyton reported his work, published in a paper called "A Concept of Negative Interstitial Pressure Based on Pressures in Implanted Perforated Capsules" that appeared in the journal *Circulation Research* in 1963.

Dr. John Hall, Guyton's successor as chairman who came to the Medical Center as a postdoctoral fellow in the physiology department, vividly remembers the antipathy this theory aroused among scientists. As a graduate student at Michigan State University, Hall gave a lecture on the negative pressure of the interstitium based on his reading and understanding of Guyton's work. "I was almost hooted down, and my chairman wasn't impressed. But Guyton was right. I don't think too many people question it now."

With all the work in cardiac output and venous return, the tissue regulation of local blood flow, and the interstitial fluid, Guyton had not forgotten his original, what he called his "ever-glorious" goal of finding out what controlled blood pressure. "The goals of youth are rarely forgotten," he said.

The turning point came in 1966 when the department had one of its early analog computers. Guyton wanted a computer model to show the effect of an increase in fluid volume on blood pressure. He had predicted that the transfusion of extra fluid volume into the "circulatory system" of the computer model would cause an initial rise in pressure that would then fall back part way toward normal. But what the model demonstrated was that the pressure fell all the way back to normal after an initial rise. Guyton had the sudden realization that "all of us, the entire physiological community had been extremely sloppy in our thinking about the role of fluid volume in the long-term regulation of arterial pressure, especially the role of the body fluids in hypertension. Furthermore, this simple computer result provided the unifying principle of arterial pressure control that we had been searching for."

What the model told them was that an increase in body fluid can cause a rise in blood pressure, but the increased pressure will then force the kidney to excrete more salt and water until the pressure returns to normal. "The discovery that the kidneys play an absolutely central role in all mechanisms of long-term pressure control was really very revolutionary even though it appears to be a very commonplace idea," Guyton wrote. "The reason it was so important was that it allowed us to concentrate on studying those factors that affect the long-term capability of the kidneys to excrete water and salt at different arterial pressure levels."

This led to an *infinite gain* theory that said that one system—fluid volume control by the kidney—could be so powerful as a long-term regulator of blood pressure that other systems can only regulate pressure short-term and will eventually be overpowered by the key controller, the kidney.

That theory, too, flew in the face of what was then the accepted notion of what causes high blood pressure—the *mosaic* theory. According to Dr. Tom Coleman, now professor emeritus of physiology who was still a graduate student when he worked with Guyton on the model, described the mosaic theory as "an incredibly complicated explanation" that included every known factor in blood pressure control. "It was then the best, the safest explanation because it couldn't be proved or disproved." It said, really, that many factors cause hypertension because there are many factors that control blood pressure. Guyton had reduced the complicated to the simple, and most of his colleagues weren't ready for the simple explanation.

When Guyton said he was lucky to enter the cardiovascular research field when he did, there may have been some happy coincidences that led to his success, but only Arthur Guyton would have considered it "luck." He directed his lifelong interest and adeptness at mathematics to electronic circuits when he was still in high school. That self-imposed independent study was crucial in the development of his thinking about ways to study body functions. The mathematical analysis of electronic systems was just beginning to be taught in engineering schools in the 1930s and, Guyton said, the mathematical analysis of electrical circuits is exactly the same as the mathematical analysis of the circulatory system. When he started in the field of cardiovascular physiology, he said most physiologists were trained as biologists. Very few had mathematical or physics training. What that led to was a science filled with verbal descriptions of complex body functions. Guyton and his students changed all that. Physiology became a quantitative rather than a descriptive science. "Language gives equal value to every description. Mathematics shows what is most important," he said.

Before the advent of computers, Guyton demonstrated the mathematical formulas for various body functions on graphs. Even before his textbook was published, he used graphs in the notes he gave to students. In a sense he waited for technology to catch up with him. Dr. Tom Milhorn, who came to the Medical Center in 1960 as a physiology graduate student, worked with Guyton on his early computer models. He recalled using the digital computer that belonged to the School of Engineering at Ole Miss before the Medical Center had a computer. "The first analog computer the department had came in a kit and took up the space of half a desk top. It really just wasn't adequate to do what we needed to do," Milhorn said.

Dr. Tom Coleman, professor emeritus of physiology, came to the Medical Center as a graduate student in physiology in 1964. By this time, the department had secured funds to buy another analog computer, much bigger and more powerful than the original "kit" computer. "All of the original simulations of cardiovascular function were done on the analog computer," Coleman said. He programmed them by plugging hundreds of short jumper wires into one-foot square boards. The wires connected electrical elements that performed math functions. It was this early model that led Guyton and Coleman to understand how important the kidney was in blood pressure control. "We had always known that fluid was important, but this model showed us that it was the most important factor," Guyton said.

Coleman said from the first, they realized this model had certain very peculiar characteristics. "We couldn't change blood pressure unless we changed kidney function or changed the continuous rate of fluid intake. You could do lots of things to it and watch it respond, but blood pressure wouldn't change appreciably or for any length of time. But especially when you changed kidney function, the blood pressure changed and nothing else you could do would prevent it. It clearly demonstrated how exquisitely important the kidney was."

In 1967, when the department received the first big "program" grant from the National Institutes of Health, a state-of-the-art digital computer replaced the, by now, obsolete analog computer. In 1974, a DEC PDP-1170 replaced the 1967 model. The new model was ten times more powerful but occupied the same amount of space. Dr. Davis Manning, professor in the department, said the computer company configured this computer with the specific capability of running Guyton's large model. It occupied a big "computer room at the end of one hall." In 1987, computer technology, still packing as much or more power in smaller and smaller boxes, led to the dismantling of the once awesome PDP-1170.

Milhorn recalled how Guyton arrived at his large circulatory model on the digital computer. "He basically sat in his office and wrote out all the equations, hundreds of them. He got a book on Fortran programming and read that; he read the instruction manual that came with the computer. He programmed it all and went and put it on the computer and got it working. To the best of my knowledge, that was the first digital computer he ever touched—which was absolutely remarkable."

Dr. Allen Cowley, who came in 1968 as a postdoctoral fellow, joined the faculty and left in 1980 to become chairman of physiology at the Medical College of Wisconsin. He recalled the model's influence at a reunion of Guyton trainees. "Around the world people were finding that the model was accurately predicting the outcome of experiments. I have yet to find an instance where these predictions were wrong. Guyton, much to the chagrin of the rest of the world, had found a way to express all the factors related to arterial pressure."

The original cardiovascular system model with some four hundred equations grew constantly as more information from animal studies was added to it. The model also served a valuable function in avoiding unnecessary animal studies. As Dr. Tom Lohmeier, professor in the department, said, "An investigator could spend years working on a totally insignificant event. But the computer model helps us avoid that."

The work that Coleman and Dr. Richard Summers, professor of emergency medicine, now do with the National Aeronautics and Space Administration (NASA) to determine ways to counter the effects of weightlessness on astronauts, uses a descendent of the department's original model of the cardiovascular system.

In the mid-1970s, when the Medical Center's physiology department had a worldwide reputation for using computer models in physiology research, the department hosted an international meeting of prominent scientists from many countries who wanted to learn more about what Guyton and his colleagues were doing. Instead of a nicely catered lunch that the department could have well afforded, those gathered barely stopped from their lectures long enough to grab a packaged tuna sandwich from the cafeteria and a soft drink from a cooler.

It was typical of the austerity in which Guyton went about his work. He grew up during the depression, when Mississippi—poor to begin with—was desperately so in the national economic downturn. And even after the depression, the medical school never had budget money to spare. The new Medical Center, operating mostly on legislative appropriations, was too young to have much of an endowment of any kind.

His office in 2003 was the same as it was in 1955—metal desks, straight-backed chairs, a wooden cabinet that belonged to his father, Venetian blinds the same age as the original Medical Center building, a wall of books, and a floor of gray linoleum. When his secretary asked for a new chair, he asked her if it was the oldest chair in the department, and if it was he would replace it.

Early graduate students had to build their own equipment, learn to blow glass, and work in the machine shop. They re-used cotton as sponges in animal surgery, carefully washing, sterilizing, and drying the wads after each procedure.

His zeal for research and teaching made up for his lack of interest in the way things looked. Dr. David Young, professor emeritus of physiology, described one of Guyton's most endearing attributes as the ability to "share the joy of research. He loves science and he loves teaching, and there's no substitute for the combination."

He was also an exacting taskmaster. He worked hard, and he expected the same from his faculty. Elvin Smith recalled that Guyton spent hours working in his office, but always seemed to know, "much to the consternation of everyone, details of all the activities within the department." According to Smith, Guyton had some reason to believe that some of his employees weren't working very hard when he had to be away from the Medical Center for a speaking engagement. Guyton realized that everyone knew of his impending absence by the airline ticket folder he carried in his shirt pocket the day of his departure. "In typical Guyton fashion, he quickly devised a solution. He obtained an extra ticket folder. It became an indispensable part of his regular apparel. From that day forward he had a ticket folder in his shirt pocket whether he was going out of town or not."

He did work hard. It was a work ethic inherited from his parents. But much of what would be work to most of us, was pure enjoyment to him. His faculty members and former students all agree that their mentor was happiest when they brought him unexpected data that added an important piece to puzzle. "Sometimes we didn't know how important it was," recalled Elvin Smith. At the Jackson Cardiovascular-Renal Research Meeting 2000, a gathering of scientists who came to share their research and to honor Guyton at the time the tenth edition of his textbook was published, the honoree received three standing ovations. Then confined to a wheelchair, he held the microphone close so there would be no trouble understanding him.

"When I was on crutches, and not in this wheelchair, I was able to come to many of your departments," he told the audience that was made up of many of his former students who were now department chairs. "It was such fun, wasn't it, when we learned something most people didn't know?"

Despite failing health and a growing frailty, Guyton came to the Medical Center for four hours five days a week after his official retirement, still having fun. He still worked on his book with the assistance of Dr. John Hall, his successor, and still wrote journal articles and, no doubt, still had ideas for research. His work ended with his death, not his retirement.

Of all the people who have ever been associated with the Medical Center, no one could have left a bigger void at death. At the funeral for Guyton on April 6, 2003, at the Oxford University Methodist Church, the Medical Center's then vice chancellor Dr. Wallace Conerly expressed the great emptiness felt by Guyton's friends and colleagues at the Medical Center. The sense of loss "feels like a vast hole in the universe. Arthur Guyton's absence will be comparable in size to his presence, which was huge." He asked the question, "How do we honor the Guyton legacy while we deal with this great sense of loss?" And answered, "We can be grateful for his gifts to us and to the world. And we can do our best to follow his example of personal integrity, hard work, diligent study, and dogged persistence. And if enough of us do this, perhaps this darkness we feel now will begin to fill with light."

CHAPTER 5

Taking Down Barriers

The 1960s in Mississippi was a dismal decade. White demagogues controlled state politics, and segregation of the races was rigidly enforced if not by police action, then by common assent. Only 6 percent of African Americans of voting age in Mississippi were registered to vote before the passage of the 1965 voting rights bill, compared to 39 percent in Georgia, a state with a similar black/white population ratio. The riots on the Ole Miss campus in 1962 when James Meredith broke the color barrier at Ole Miss became the defining moment in Mississippi history for the next four decades. Nothing was the same afterward. Mississippi's collective schizophrenia was on public display. As Walker Percy noted in his 1965 essay, "Mississippi: The Fallen Paradise,"

> The rift in its [Mississippi's] character between a genuine kindliness and a highly developed individual moral consciousness on the one hand and on the other a purely political and amoral view of "states' rights" at the expense of human rights led at last to a sundering of its very soul.

Things would get worse after the Ole Miss riots, not better. The civil rights leader Medgar Evers would be murdered in Jackson in 1963, and three freedom riders would be murdered in Philadelphia in 1964. There was hardly any good news coming out of Mississippi in the 1960s. The national press, understandably caught up in the drama of evil, overlooked many acts of bravery and opposition to prevailing policies. The one bright spot—ironically recognized by segregationists and their opposites alike—was the University of Mississippi Medical Center. When Dean David Pankratz resigned early in February of 1961, the Medical Center was six years old and full of optimism. Its faculty was making national headlines and getting national awards. Grants for research were plentiful, and public support was high.

A January 19, 1961, article in the Jackson *State Times* hailed the Medical Center's successful use of electrical anesthesia, which had received national media coverage, as "the most important medical discovery ever made in Mississippi." (In later years, despite its promise and the interest it aroused in the lay press, the program was dropped. A key engineer was recruited by the private sector before the research could prove it to be a viable alternative to existing anesthesia.) On February 16, 1962, the Jackson *Clarion-Ledger* printed a feature from the Medical Center's public affairs office that described key work in the basic science departments for which investigators had won awards and received substantial grant support. The article described the transplantation of hearts in dogs, the physiology department's work in cardiac output, and the microbiology department's study of viruses that may lead to cancer (then a new concept) and studies of the immune system. Showing its support for the Medical Center's promise as an important research institution, the Mississippi Legislature had approved a $1 million appropriation to match a federal source of $2 million to build the research wing, the first major addition onto the original complex.

The appointment of Dr. Robert Q. Marston in July of 1961 as dean of the medical school and director of the Medical Center seemed to be the zenith of that optimism—the bright reward for the hard work and dedication of so many of the Medical Center's first family. Marston proved equal to his promise. He was adept at securing funding from the legislature, and he helped deliver the institution through the bitter years of the turbulent sixties. He managed to walk the tightrope over political chasms that had potentially devastating consequences for the Medical Center if he lost his footing.

Marston was a native Virginian, a graduate of the Virginia Military Institute and the Medical College of Virginia. He did postgraduate training in prominent southern medical centers, Johns Hopkins University Hospital, Vanderbilt University, and the Medical College of Virginia. He was also a Rhodes scholar at Oxford University. He was a Markle Scholar in Medicine under a program the Markle Foundation established in 1947 "in response to a need for more teachers, researchers and administrators in the nation's medical schools." The program awarded grants to gifted practitioners planning to further their career in academic medicine. Before coming to Mississippi, Marston had been on the faculty at the Medical College of Virginia and the University of Minnesota.

He was thirty-eight at the time of his appointment in Jackson, and a reporter for the Jackson *State Times* called him "a slim young man who emanates self-assurance and ability." According to Maurine Twiss, the director of public information at the Medical Center, Marston was handsome and charming, and he used both attributes to the Medical Center's advantage. He also came, if not with a clear mandate, then with the certain understanding that he would facilitate the orderly integration of the Medical Center. Marston said he told the university chancellor

J. D. Williams that he was in favor of integration while the chancellor was interviewing him for the job in Mississippi. According to Marston, Williams told him, "I do not think we would be talking to you if you were not."

Marston's tenure began about a year before the University of Mississippi in Oxford was forced to enroll its first black student, James Meredith. The riot that ensued left two dead and many more wounded. Two years into his post, on June 11, 1963, the civil rights leader Medgar Evers was murdered on the same night Dr. James Hardy, chairman of surgery at the Medical Center, performed the world's first lung transplant. Evers, in fact, was brought to the Medical Center's emergency room where a member of Hardy's transplant team, Dr. Martin Dalton, left Hardy's side to rush to the ER where his resuscitation efforts failed. In the summer of 1964, the bodies of three young men who came to Mississippi to help black Mississippians register to vote were found buried in Neshoba County, the victims of murder. Their bodies came to the Medical Center for autopsies, and with them came a host of national media representatives and members of numerous civil rights organizations, all angry. It was the same summer that President Lyndon Johnson signed the civil rights law into effect guaranteeing all citizens equal access to employment and education without regard to race.

During this tumultuous period in Mississippi's history, the state's only Medical Center had to appease two masters with diametrically opposing demands. In 1956, a group of state legislators reported that it had halted "creeping racial integration" in the new University Hospital by making the hospital discontinue the mixing of black and white employees during orientation. As late as 1962 the Mississippi Legislature investigated the Medical Center for allowing black and white children to play and watch television together. In defiance of national standards and laws, Mississippi's government justified its actions on the basis of its rights as a sovereign state. To Marston's everlasting credit, he managed to assuage the fears of the staunchest segregationists in state government while never giving in on what he knew had to be done to comply with federal mandates.

M. M. Roberts, a member of the Board of Trustees, Institutions of Higher Learning, was a staunch supporter of segregationist governor Ross Barnett and believed fervently in states' rights and in segregation. Yet, as Twiss recalled, his response to Marston's requests was usually, "I will do whatever he says must be done." Marston, who died in 1999, recounted some of his experiences in Mississippi during a 1988 interview for the Samuel Proctor Oral History Project of the University of Florida. Marston recalled that he and Roberts were together on a small plane making a tour of state facilities where they discussed each other's views on a number of topics.

The press was waiting when they got off the plane, and reporters began asking Roberts about their conversation. According to Marston, Roberts told the reporters, "We disagreed on everything we discussed but he is doing a good job for that Medical Center and I am going to support him because of the importance of the Medical Center to the state of Mississippi."

The Medical Center, unlike its parent campus, never experienced a violent reaction to its attempts to obey federal law. Integration was accomplished quietly and with no fanfare. Timing was on its side because when integration happened, it was already the law of the land. By 1965, state officials knew that resistence was futile. It may also have been because the Medical Center, new and businesslike, was not the mythic symbol of the Old South that Ole Miss was. The general public's attachment to the Medical Center was practical, not emotional. And many Mississippi legislators, as well as board officials such as Roberts, who fought so hard to keep Meredith out of Ole Miss, were willing to suspend their concern with "federal encroachment" when it came to the Medical Center.

The IHL board, Governor Ross Barnett, and university officials had used every means at their disposal to defy the U.S. Supreme Court order to admit Meredith to the university. But the actions of the board and the riots on the Oxford campus had only a peripheral effect on the Medical Center. At one point, Marston told a group of agitated medical students that if they went to Oxford they would not be excused from classes and reminded them that their first duty was to their patients. None, as far as Marston knew, participated in the riots in Oxford. The IHL board used Marston's conference room at the Medical Center in the weeks immediately preceding Meredith's enrollment (October 1, 1962) when board members wanted to go into executive session.

Dr. Verner Holmes, the ENT surgeon from McComb, was in his first twelve-year term on the board. He called the five-hour meeting in Marston's conference room on September 19, 1962, the "worst experience of the whole time." Opinion on the board was sharply divided on whether to admit Meredith and comply with Supreme Court orders. Six, including Holmes and Tally Riddell, favored compliance over contempt of court charges. It was Holmes, in fact, who two days earlier had told a reporter that he would not go to jail and would not vote to close Ole Miss. Barnett's appointees on the board had said they would close the university and go to jail if necessary to keep Meredith out.

This sharp division and the presence of a governor running out of options set the tension level for the meeting on September 19. Apparently discussion got so heated that Tally Riddell had to be admitted to University Hospital that night, ostensibly from the strain on his heart brought on by the stress of the meeting. Riddell, however, told Marston, who checked on him the next day, that he had feigned a heart attack. He told Marston that the governor became so verbally abusive that Riddell drew back his fist and was about to sock the governor when rational thought held sway. Riddell said he suddenly had the sobering thought that he was a split second away from assaulting the governor of Mississippi.

The Medical Center again faced the threat of losing its accreditation if the Southern Association of Colleges and Schools pulled the University of Mississippi from its list of accredited institutions. At one point, the IHL board had appointed Barnett registrar of the university so that he personally would have the responsibility for Meredith's enrollment. SACS saw this as political interference with the governance of an institution of higher learning, the same issue that got the universities in trouble in the 1930s when Governor Theodore Bilbo began hiring and firing administrators and faculty at the state's universities. If the parent institution lost its accreditation with SACS, the agencies that accredit medical schools would have certainly followed suit. But the board quickly rescinded Barnett's appointment as registrar very soon after the riots, so accreditation was maintained.

In the summer of 1964, Mississippi was a battleground in the struggle for black equality. Freedom Riders from the north, idealistic young college students for the most part, poured into Mississippi for voter registration drives. The violent opposition of the Ku Klux Klan, or government-sanctioned opposition like the Mississippi Sovereignty Commission, tried to thwart their activities wherever possible, either by violence or by selective enforcement of local laws. Michael Schwerner, Andrew Goodman, and James Chaney, all members of the Congress of Racial Equality (CORE) were reported missing on June 21 or 22, after they had been arrested by Neshoba County deputy sheriff Cecil Price. Their bodies were found in a dam near Philadelphia on August 4, 1964. Klansmen admitted to participating in and witnessing the murder. The Federal Bureau of Investigation (FBI) mounted an extensive investigation and ordered the bodies taken to the Medical Center for autopsy. They arrived just after midnight on August 5. Dr. Joel Brunson, chairman of pathology, Dr. John Gronvall, a pathologist whom Marston had appointed to be his right-hand man, and Dr. William Featherston, a pathologist in private practice in Jackson, all did the autopsies, access to which was carefully controlled by the FBI. Maurine Twiss recalled that at least a day or two later, Dr. David Spain, a pathologist at the Brookdale Medical Center in Brooklyn, New York, performed a second autopsy on Schwerner and Chaney at the request of their parents. After doing the autopsies, in the presence of Brunson, Gronvall, and Featherston, he charged that the first pathology report was false. According to Twiss, there was no pathology report on the autopsies on the orders of the FBI, whose investigators were building their case. "The FBI's statement merely said the three had been shot. Spain said they'd been beaten, which no one had ever denied. Spain implied in his statement that the Medical Center, the university, had been part of a coverup." Spain later wrote a first-person account of his trip to Mississippi that was published in the magazine *Ramparts*, in which he likened Mississippi physicians to those in Nazi Germany. He implied that the Medical Center faculty was in league with the murderers and that incomplete information about the autopsies was released by the Medical Center. The allegations, all untrue, would probably have done no harm if that were the end of it. Few physicians or scientists read *Ramparts* for the veracity of its science reporting. But Dr. Louis Lasagna, associate professor of medicine at Johns Hopkins, gave a lecture on "Mind and Morality of the Doctor" at the 1965 Yale Lectures on Medical Ethics. He quoted extensively and verbatim from Spain's first-person account, and his lecture was subsequently published in the Yale *Journal of Biology and Medicine*. "He had tied us all up in a bundle, Mississippi and Nazi Germany," Twiss recalled. "And now that the allegations were in a reputable scientific journal we could no longer ignore them." Marston wrote a letter in rebuttal, which the journal printed, but according to Twiss, the inflammatory language, the unsubstantiated charges, once in print, "had a lingering long-term effect on the perception of people who mattered to us. It cast a shadow over the Medical Center which loomed there for a long time."

The Philadelphia killings preceded by one month the signing of the landmark civil rights law by President Lyndon Johnson. The worst of the violence was over, but it would be difficult to measure how the events of 1962, 1963, and 1964 affected life at the Medical Center. Certainly recruiting from out of state was made much more difficult. "Sometimes the husband would agree to come for a visit, but his wife would be afraid to get off the plane," Twiss recalled. And the distrust of Mississippians away from home was palpable. "When we went to meetings in large hotels, bell hops would refuse to carry our bags," James Hardy recounted in his memoirs. Dr. Blair Batson, the chairman of pediatrics, recalled how a pediatrician from Boston "lit into" him at a big meeting after the Philadelphia murders. Dr. Robert Currier, the chairman of the Department of Neurology, described the mood of the Medical Center faculty as "being under seige" and at the mercy of whatever political force was paramount. It was not a time that could be characterized as conducive to extraordinary work, but interestingly enough, the years of 1960–1965 were among the most noteworthy of any five-year period in the Medical Center's history.

When Robert Marston recalled his career in academic medicine, he said that he was fortunate to have been in positions when it was possible to influence the course of history, and that was certainly where he found himself in Mississippi. It could be argued that all the changes made by the Medical Center could have been accomplished under any leadership because they were mandated by the federal government, specifically by the civil rights legislation passed in 1964. Had the Medical Center failed to obey the law, it would have lost research funds, training grants, and money for physical facilities appropriated by a Congress eager to see a national system of first-rate medical education and research centers. And yet, Marston has to be credited with such a smooth transition into the era of equal rights. Marston said it was his intention to integrate the Medical Center from the very beginning of his tenure, and that the civil rights legislation in 1964 gave him the authority to do so. In fact, he said the original blueprints for the Medical Center did not accommodate segregation. It was designed for the future, for a time when segregation would sound like a horrifying custom.

On January 13, 1965, at an administrative staff meeting, Marston described the four reasons for the meeting: to make sure everyone was familiar with the civil rights legislation that President Lyndon Johnson had signed in July 1964 and that went into effect on January 3, 1965; to state the Medical Center's intention to comply with the law; to identify areas in which changes would be necessary; and to seek methods and initiate action to ensure compliance. Maurine Twiss, director of public affairs at the time, recalled that she "leaked" an item to the local press about the meeting. The *Jackson Daily News* dutifully printed the quote from the weekly calendar at the Medical Center, that steps were being taken "without unnecessary delay or unworkable haste" to comply with the Civil Rights Act of 1964. The phrase "unworkable haste" proved to be prophetic.

Marston had already removed the "white" and "colored" signs over water fountains and restrooms and combined the "white" and "colored" sections of the cafeteria upon the advice of the university attorney J. D. Doty. After reviewing the forms from the President's Committee on Equal Employment Opportunity that Marston signed on July 2, 1964, Doty advised Marston that the Medical Center must be able to answer "no" to the question, "Are there any employee facilities which are provided for employees on a racially segregated basis?" to be in compliance. Twiss recalled that the physical plant director, Ted Waldrom, asked that his staff not be asked to remove the signs because some of them had strong feelings in the matter. His department was one of the few at the Medical Center that had black employees at the time. In a 1963 report on employment by race, the Medical Center employed

133 black males, 116 of whom were "service workers." Of the 190 black women employed, 137 were in the same category. Instead of forcing the issue, Marston used his administrative team to take down most of the "white" and "colored" signs during the course of one night. "Having little time to prepare for this, we had gotten case knives from the cafeteria to take down the signs," Twiss said. Marston said that months later, after he had enlisted the help of some black physicians to help the Medical Center face its compliance issues, they brought him signs, one "white," one "colored," that had been missed the first time. He said they told him that blacks knew where all the signs were, even the ones that had been hidden for years on doors that had never been closed. He kept the "colored" sign in his office during his decade at the University of Florida as a memento of his Mississippi years. The "white" sign he gave to his old friend and colleague Dr. Verner Holmes.

Around the same time, Marston asked architect Todd Wheeler how the cafeteria could be opened up so it would no longer be segregated by color. Wheeler found that the wall was not weight bearing and said the whole wall could be removed, which was done.

In February of 1965, "This Week at UMC," the weekly calendar of events for the Medical Center, announced that the hospital would begin moving patients to comply with the civil rights law, putting all surgery patients on one floor and all medical patients on another floor without regard to race. At this time, neither Marston nor any of his administrative staff had any inkling about how the new law was going to be enforced. By calling every federal agency that the Medical Center thought might have information, officials finally, on March 1, came up with a checklist that investigators would use in deciding compliance. It was mostly concerned with the integration of hospital facilities, both inpatient and outpatient, and the integration of the medical staff. On March 5, the Associated Press released the story about the National Association for the Advancement of Colored People (NAACP) filing complaints against twenty-nine hospitals, including the University Hospital in Jackson. A month later, Marston and his staff were still trying to discover what charges had been filed against the hospital and to what federal agency should they answer. Their quandary reflected Washington's disarray in the whole matter. From agency to agency, there was no clear understanding about how to proceed. In a letter to Dr. Roger B. Arhelger, assistant professor of pathology at the Medical Center, then vice president Hubert Humphrey declared, "Passage of the 1964 civil rights act has imposed upon the Federal government a tremendous responsibility and a heavy administrative burden. To be perfectly candid, it will take some time and additional experience before we can meet this administrative challenge as effectively as we would all wish; in the interim, we are indeed grateful for the understanding and cooperation given by thoughtful and sincere individuals like Dr. Marston."

While still not knowing what the charges were, Marston told a meeting of the South Central Medical Society on March 9 that complaints will be filed against the Medical Center and that when "requirements for compliance are spelled out, we will meet them." Marston said in that speech, "I have heard recently that the Medical Center has been accused of moving too rapidly; of becoming too integrated. Obviously, this is untrue. I am further deeply concerned and disappointed to hear that people are using this untruth to weaken and undermine the Center. The Medical Center is a creation of the people of the State of Mississippi and of the medical profession in the state. It can be destroyed or harmed most quickly not by those outside of the state but by the same people who created it. The center needs your support and help as never before." On March 11, the chairman of pharmacology, Dr. William Holland, offered a faculty position to Dr. Marion Myles. She accepted the offer on March 13 and agreed to start work on June 1—the Medical Center's first black faculty member. Maurine Twiss recalled that Marston had been "casting about for a black faculty member for some time . . . and Bill Holland came up with Marion Myles."

Myles was an assistant professor of pharmacology who studied the effects of drugs and hormones on plant growth. She was born in Philadelphia and was graduated from the University of Pennsylvania. She earned the PhD at Iowa State University and did postdoctoral training at the California Institute of Technology, Oak Ridge Institute of Nuclear Studies, Iowa State University of Science and Technology, the University of Tennessee, and Vanderbilt University. She was teaching at Alcorn A & M when she was recruited by Holland. She stayed at the Medical Center until her death in 1969.

On April 12, Twiss said they heard unofficially that grant support would be withheld from institutions charged with discrimination, but again they failed to get any information from either the Public Health Service or the Department of Health, Education, and Welfare (DHEW). "At that point, we knew we had to do something even it were wrong," Maurine Twiss recalled. "That very night we began marathon meetings that didn't end until after the April 16 inspection."

On April 13, Marston made the bold move of telling James Quigley, assistant secretary of the DHEW, that the Medical Center was ready for an inspection. According to both Twiss and Marston, Marston insisted that Quigley send the toughest inspector the department had. "Anyone from the Atlanta office will be suspect. I want someone from Washington," Marston told Quigley, who assured Marston that the Medical Center would get their most formidable inspector, Sherry Arnstein. According to Marston, Quigley told him, "She tells me that if she comes to Mississippi and finds the Medical Center in compliance, she'll begin her report with 'Christ has risen again.'"

Much to the surprise of everyone at the Medical Center, who thought they would have several weeks to get ready for an inspection, Quigley assigned Sherry Arnstein and William Burleigh to be at the Medical Center on April 16. That gave the Medical Center forty-eight hours to get ready. Marston had forced the issue, much to his credit in the eyes of the inspection team, but harrowing to the administrative team. Marston gave hospital director Dr. David Wilson further instruction on integrating the patient population, making sure that white patients and black patients were on the same floor, that white patients and black patients occupied four-bed units together. Although integration of patients had begun in March when students were on spring break, the shuffling of patients on April 15 represented the most extensive integration of patients yet. "None of the patients who had to be moved that night expressed any objection at all," Twiss recalled.

When Arnstein and Burleigh completed their inspection, Twiss said they left, pleased with the state of integration at the Medical Center and with only two areas of concern, ob-gyn and psychiatry. They left with the assurance that additional changes would be made. On May 28, the Medical Center was officially cleared of all charges of discrimination, becoming one of only a dozen that "satisfied us with their corrective actions," Quigley was quoted as saying. It was also the first of twenty-nine medical centers to be inspected. It took another month for word to get through to all the federal granting agencies that the Medical Center was in compliance, and there was a brief period in which grant recipients received frightening letters telling them their grants would be held until their institution met federal guidelines.

Apparently Arnstein was true to her word and began her report, "Christ has risen again." According to Marston, who met her thirty years later at a meeting in Washington, she introduced herself and said, "You probably don't remember me." To which he replied, "Of course I do. You're the lady who starts her reports, 'Christ has risen again.'"

Meanwhile, Marston was in a silent struggle with the IHL board, who had refused to move on the appointment of Myles, the first black faculty member. Marston had recommended her to the board at its March 25 meeting, but it was now May 21 and the board had not acted on the recommendation. A lot hinged on her appointment. Marston had let Quigley know in April that he had hired a black faculty member. The Medical Center needed proof that it was in compliance both with the letter and spirit of the civil rights law. He wrote to Verner Holmes, by then chairman of the IHL board and still a stalwart friend of the Medical Center, outlining the guidelines and laws on civil rights that pertained to the facility and the actions it had taken to comply with the laws. "The fact that this action [contract with Myles] had been taken was undoubtedly a key point in our attempts to have the University Hospital cleared of charges of discrimination. I have been asked repeatedly by Mr. James M. Quigley, assistant secretary of the Department of Health, Education, and Welfare, and others, what evidence we have of nondiscrimination in the selection of students and faculty members. This appointment is the single example which we could submit." Marston also told Twiss that he told E. R. Jobe, the executive director of the board, that he was going to hire Myles unless he heard a no from Jobe. Twiss maintained that Jobe knew he couldn't say "do it" without a vote of the board, but he also knew that if he said nothing, Marston would take it as assent. Then with Marston's letter in hand, Holmes "browbeat or shamed the board into finally taking action." Myles began her job on July 1.

Quigley had told Marston that the Medical Center's successful inspection was not the end, merely the beginning, as indeed it was. Inspectors continued to point out that the cafeteria remained segregated despite the removal of the wall. Integration began to occur more frequently when Marston ordered the second line closed. Compliance with federal law required reams of documentation over the course of many years and careful adherence to education and employment regulations.

Marston had made an impression with his handling of the Medical Center's compliance. In 1966, he was appointed associate director of the National Institutes of Health in charge of the new federal initiative, the Regional Medical Program, to attack the three major killers of Americans—heart disease, cancer, and stroke. In 1968, he was named director of NIH. Marston was abruptly dismissed from his post after criticizing President Richard Nixon's declaration of "war on cancer" for the damage he thought it did to other research initiatives. He was scholar in residence at the University of Virginia from 1973 until 1974, and served as president of the University of Florida from 1974 until 1984. Marston died in 1999 at the age of seventy-six.

The chancellor added "vice chancellor" to Marston's title in 1965, a designation that would not be made again until Norman Nelson's appointment in 1973. Marston's assistant dean, Dr. John Gronvall, served as interim director of the Medical Center for one year until the appointment of Dr. Robert Carter in 1967 as dean of the medical school and director of the Medical Center. Carter was associate dean of the School of Medicine and professor of pediatrics at the Iowa

College of Medicine in Iowa City when he was tapped for the Mississippi post. He had received both his BS and MD from the University of Minnesota, interned at Cleveland City Hospital, and took his pediatric residency at the University of Chicago where he served on the faculty from 1956 to 1959. He was also a staff member and associate group leader at the Los Alamos Scientific Laboratory of the University of California for three years where he investigated the effects of radiation. It was Carter who designed the County Health Improvement Project in Holmes County, the precursor the highly acclaimed nurse midwifery program.

By 1969, the Office for Civil Rights out of the Department of Health, Education, and Welfare was the channel through which the Medical Center worked in meeting federal standards. An inspection by DHEW in December of 1968 found the Medical Center "out of compliance" with civil rights laws. The report noted "some positive steps taken," including "your efforts through a biracial council to make contact with the leadership of the minority group community, several instances in which Negro employees are in a supervisory position and the presence on your full time faculty of one Negro with professorial responsibilities." The report, however, urged a more aggressive approach at recruiting. Predominantly black high schools and colleges should be urged by the Medical Center to have a team visit their campus. Advertising for positions should include a rigorous search for publications with black readership. The report further stated, "Although it was apparent that neither of the schools [nursing or medicine] has actively sought to discourage the admission or involvement of Negro students, it is in the area of affirmative action that we have some concerns about the compliance status." The Medical Center prepared a plan addressing the long list of suggestions by the inspection team, and the plan was approved in April of 1970 by Horace A. Bohannon, the acting regional civil rights director for DHEW.

Carter left in 1970, succeeded by Dr. Robert E. Blount, who had come to the Medical Center in 1968 after his retirement from the army at the rank of major general. His last military post was as commanding officer at Fitzsimons Hospital in Denver, Colorado. Blount's distinguished military career took him to the Philippines and Europe during World War II and to assignments at Walter Reed and Brooke General Hospitals in peace time. Carter had named Blount the institution's equal opportunity officer when Blount was assistant dean in 1969. After Blount became dean, he appointed Dr. Robert D. Sloan, chairman of radiology, to chair a committee charged with minority enrollment.

The recruitment of African American students and faculty at the Medical Center was accomplished in fits and starts. It was complicated by the fact that public academic institutions all over the country faced the same compliance issues as the Medical Center. Mississippi was competing with institutions who could offer qualified black students irresistible financial packages to boost their minority enrollment. Also, the Medical Center was slow to adopt the posture of aggressive minority recruitment.

The first black resident was Dr. Aaron Shirley, now chairman of the Jackson Medical Mall Foundation and director of the Medical Center's community outreach services. He had gone to medical school at Meharry Medical College in Nashville, Tennessee, with tuition assistance from the IHL board. To avoid integration, the board had established a program that paid tuition for African American students in Mississippi to attend professional schools out of state. In return, the students were obligated to spend five years practicing in Mississippi. "I always wanted to be a pediatrician, so from day one, it was my plan to work five years and then get out of Mississippi to do a pediatric residency," Shirley said. So in 1960, Shirley was in Vicksburg to begin his five-year obligatory service to a state that paid for his education, but did not want to train him as a physician. Shirley opened his private practice but found himself with no hospital to refer his patients to in Vicksburg. "None would give me admitting privileges. If I had a patient that needed hospitalization, I had to refer them to University Hospital." In doing so, he established a relationship with the Medical Center's Department of Pediatrics, especially with Dr. David Watson, the pediatric cardiologist.

In 1964, toward the end of his five-year commitment, he applied for a residency in pediatrics to the University of Oklahoma and to the University of Mississippi Medical Center. "Oklahoma was my real choice; I applied to the Medical Center out of curiosity more than anything else. My wife's grandparents were in Oklahoma, and things weren't as bad for blacks there." Oklahoma, however, did not have a slot available starting in July 1965, but offered him a slot in 1966. To Shirley's great surprise, Dr. Blair Batson called him to discuss his application for the residency in Jackson. They met for an interview, and Batson called him a week later to tell him that a slot would open up in November 1965 if he was interested. "I told him I'd have to think about it, but after my wife and I discussed it, we decided to stay here and try to make a difference." Because of his five years in practice before he started his residency, Shirley was given a year's credit toward his residency requirement so the usual three-year residency period was reduced to two for him.

"Dr. Batson made it clear to the physicians who admitted patients to the pediatric service, that the resident was in charge, so none of the referring physicians who were white seemed to have any problem with me being there. There were a good many white patients, and I never had one white parent resist me being their child's physician." At the end of his residency in 1967, when he had other opportunities to go elsewhere, he decided to stay. He saw the sad results in children when access to health care is minimal. "I saw so many desperately ill babies who could have been managed locally and so many babies whose parents could not take the steps to get the care the child needed."

Shirley was for many years the only black pediatrician in Mississippi. He worked with the American Academy of Pediatricians as a consultant to the Head Start program and fought the attempts of two Mississippi governors to veto funding for the school readiness program.

The first black graduate student was Dr. Thomas Patterson, who earned the PhD in microbiology in 1970. The chairman of microbiology, Dr. Charles Randall, recruited Patterson from the ranks of the technicians in the department. Randall said Patterson was an army veteran who exhibited excellent work habits and intelligence. Randall said he asked Patterson if he wanted to be a graduate student. Patterson told Randall he didn't think a black man would ever have a chance to do that, and Randall told him, "Now you do." Dr. Rowe Byers, professor of microbiology, was Patterson's advisor. "He was older than most of the other students, so he was much more mature than most students. He was enormously personable and likable," Byers said. "He was just studious and hard-working. He never talked about discrimination, and I don't think he experienced any in this department." Byers said when he finished his final oral exam for his PhD, the other members in the department wanted to take him out to celebrate. Patterson declined, and Byers quoted Patterson as saying, "I just want to go somewhere and let what has happened to me happen. I need to think about it." He went on to teach at a university in Louisiana.

Sammie Inez Long was the first African American medical student. She enrolled in 1966, but withdrew in 1968. Carrie Paul Hunter was the second black medical student. She came in 1967 and transferred to New York University in 1968. The first black medical student to graduate was Dr. James Oliver, who graduated in 1972. Oliver described his years at the Medical Center in an interview with the author on May 18, 2004. "There was rarely any overt hostility. The worst time for me was when the students at Jackson State were shot by the police. I just couldn't believe that anyone could support the actions of the state troopers or the police who killed the JSU students."

Oliver bore jokes at his expense. One classmate told him he was surprised to see him in class that day because it was a black holiday, the day that General Motors runs the new Cadillacs off the assembly line. Oliver heard another joke that went around the day his lab partner choked on Oliver's blood during a demonstration for using a pipette. Tainted with black blood, the classmate went home to find a beat-up Cadillac in front of his house, his wife gone with the postman, and himself able to dance like James Brown. Laughing about it thirty-two years later, Oliver said, "The Cadillac and postman parts may ring true, but there's no way in hell he could have ever danced like James Brown."

But, he says, two or three of his classmates went out of their way to be support-ive and friendly—William Douglas Owen of Gulfport, Kelly O'Neal of Hattiesburg, and Paul William Pierce III of Vicksburg—and in spite of the jokes, he remembers his time at the Medical Center fondly. "I admit I had a chip on my shoulder. I had volunteered for military duty at the height of the Vietnam War, I had been a good citizen and felt my country owed me something. I remember sitting in class dis-cussing the war before the instructor got there. I had done my time during Viet-nam, but I was against the war. One of my classmates asked me if I was a commu-nist, and Bill [Owen] came to my defense. He said you can't call Jim a communist just because you don't agree with him."

It would probably have been better for him, he says, if there had been other black medical students. At the time, he was the only one. "Sammie [Long] was a junior when I was a freshman. We all went home for Thanksgiving, and I got a call from Sammie saying she was not coming back, that she couldn't take it any longer. I thought, 'My God, what did I get myself into.'" Dr. Richard Boronow, a member of the faculty in ob-gyn, later confided to Oliver that he thought he was perhaps the reason she withdrew because he had given her a severe dressing down for something he said she missed on a patient history. Boronow told him, "I almost got fired for it."

Oliver didn't set out to break race barriers. He only wanted to go to medical school and applied to the IHL board for tuition benefits through the same program Aaron Shirley had used to attend Meharry. He was told that since the state now had a medical school and since the enrollment was now open to blacks, the program was no longer in existence. So he applied for medical school in Mississippi.

He remembers many of his teachers as being particularly helpful—Dr. Peter Blake, Dr. Richard Boronow, Dr. Jeanette Pullen, and Dr. Herbert Langford. Langford, in fact, recommended Oliver for his internship at Boston City Hospital where he com-pleted two years of residency training and two years as a cardiology fellow. He spent seven years on the faculty at Howard University as assistant professor of medicine and director of the coronary care unit at Howard University Hospital. He's now in private practice in Washington, D.C.

Langford was Oliver's advisor as well as his physician. Oliver was diagnosed with high blood pressure during his student days, and Langford treated him. Langford probably related to Oliver's unpopular antiwar sentiments having himself been branded a communist sympathizer by a Jackson newspaper. In 1966, Tom Ethridge, a columnist for the *Clarion-Ledger*, named Langford along with William E. Holder, on the Law School faculty at Ole Miss, Russell Barrett, professor of political science at Ole Miss, Dr. David S. Lindsay, instructor in political science at the University of Southern Mississippi, and Rabbi Howard K. Kummer of Canton as signers of a petition in support of three people "whose records show they have been members of the Communist Party." One of the three was Dr. Jeremiah Stamler, one of Langford's longtime colleagues in hypertension studies. Stamler, Yolanda Farkas Hall, Stamler's assistant, and Milton M. Cohen, one of Stamler's associates, "have been active members of the Communist Party and hold key positions in their profession allegedly used to promote Red objectives," Ethridge wrote. Hundreds of academics signed the petition in support of the three, accused of "defiance, hostility and refusal to cooperate with the House Un-American Activities Committee" and threatened with contempt citations from Congress. Langford seemed not to have been bothered too much by having his association with a "known communist" recognized in print.

During medical school, Oliver also served on the Medical Center's first minority student recruitment committee, chaired by Dr. Robert Sloan, chairman of radiology. Oliver recalled that "we had a good time" during the meetings in Sloan's office. "At that time it was Dr. Sloan, Dr. Helen Barnes, Dr. Louis Sulya [chairman of biochemistry and of the medical school admissions committee] and me."

Asked if he would go through it all again, Oliver didn't hesitate to say yes. "It allowed me to fulfill my dream, and for that I will always be indebted. Oliver grew up in Hernando and graduated from Mississippi Valley State University. Mississippi is his home, and he said, if given the opportunity, he'd come back to live and practice 'in a minute.'"

Dr. Ponjola (classmates called her "P.J.") Coney, an African American, graduated from medical school in 1978, six years after Oliver got his MD. She went to the University of North Carolina at Chapel Hill for an ob-gyn residency, then was chairman of the ob-gyn department at the University of Southern Illinois. Now she is dean of the school of medicine at Meharry Medical College in Nashville, Tennessee, the first Medical Center graduate to become dean of a medical school. Coney describes her four years as a medical student as some of the best years of her life. Just twelve years after James Meredith forced Mississippi to accept black students in its colleges and universities, Coney's classmates voted her vice president of her class. She was one of 15 black students in her class of 150, and one of 28 women in her class. Gender, she remembered, was a fiercer battleground than race. Among her fellow students, she said she never "had any encounters that were hostile because of my race, and I never heard any of the other black students report any. We worked hard, interacted well, and race was not an issue." Coney says people often just don't believe her when she tells them about her medical school experience. "They say, 'you must have just missed it.'" Coney isn't an apologist for the Medical Center. There was a patient, she recalled, a wealthy farmer who came in with lung cancer. She went in to take his history, and he wouldn't talk to her and asked to be transferred to another local hospital. And once, when she asked for assistance from financial aid, she was told there was none available. At the same time, another of her male classmates reported that he had just gotten a loan from financial aid for his honeymoon. But to Coney, these incidents were of minor consequence. The major factors to her were the acceptance and respect she got from her peers and her teachers.

Coney grew up on a fifty-acre farm in Pike County, the daughter of parents who had started out as sharecroppers. One of seven children, she was the first person in her family to go to college. "I was always a good student, which was amazing considering how little I was in school. School didn't start for us until harvest was done, so sometimes I missed a good two months every year." But she learned about the world from her great-grandfather, someone who saw the budding scholar in the little girl who sat at his feet. He had college in mind for her from the very beginning. "He talked to me about everything—world events, wars, politics. He would explain how times were changing and that I should be prepared for the changes that would permit me to get an education and do great things. "

At Xavier College in New Orleans, she realized—even though she was salutatorian of her class at her high school in Magnolia—that her preparation for college was not as good as her classmates. "I had never seen a light microscope before. We had one old microscope in high school and you had to reflect the light through it. At Xavier, the lab had microscopes you could plug in, so I stayed in the lab all night trying to bring myself up to speed. I survived and thought only as far as graduating from Xavier." Her first job out of college was at the Medical Center as a medical technologist in the acute care lab. She became friends with some of the black medical students who brought specimens to the lab and talked to her while they waited for the results. "Adolf Harper was a junior at the time. He was very encouraging. He said, 'You're smart enough for medical school; you can do it.'"

She applied to Vanderbilt, Meharry, Howard, and UMC. Vanderbilt accepted her as an alternate, and she was accepted provisionally by the Mississippi medical school. "My acceptance was conditional; I had to get two more hours of physics." She reached an agreement with Mississippi College where she finished physics at night while still working in the acute lab during the day. When Coney told her parents about being accepted to medical school, she met with resistance. Having lived through the most brutal days of segregation, her parents had a difficult time believing that the culture had changed to that extent. "My mother was astonished. She said, 'they won't let you do that.' And she was genuinely frightened for me."

Coney's first day of medical school in 1974 seemed to set the tone for her next four years. She was interviewed by a reporter as a member of the largest entering medical school class in the Medical Center's history—150. A photographer took her picture, which appeared as a mug shot in the next day's paper. "One of the white male students sought me out to give me a clipping of that story. He said, 'I thought you might like to keep this.' He was William Clayton, and from day one, we became friends. We went for coffee, began talking, and talked every day for the next four years."

The recruitment of minority students began to be more systematic after the institution's plan of compliance of 1970 was approved by the DHEW. The establishment of the Office of Minority Student Affairs in 1973 helped formalize programs that would identify potential health professional students from the predominantly black colleges in the state and help them stay in school once they got here. The biggest boost to minority recruitment for the medical school came in 2000 when James and Sally Barksdale gave $2 million to the Medical Center to endow the Barksdale Scholarships. The gift made possible three full medical school scholarships per year for African American students. Each scholarship is worth approximately $22,000 a year. James Barksdale is the former CEO of Netscape. He and the late Sally Barksdale are Ole Miss alumni whose gift to the Oxford campus established the Barksdale Honors College.

In fall 2004, the Medical Center has a total enrollment in all schools of 2,005. Of those, 267 are African American. Of that 267, 29 are in medical school, 10 in dental school, 49 in nursing school, 78 in the School of Health Related Professions, 62 in the graduate school, and 33 in the residency programs. Of the 61 students in certificate programs (radiologic technology and nuclear medicine technology), 6 are African American.

In terms of equal access to health professional education, the Medical Center has made giant strides since the 1960s. But that decade, so fraught with political upheaval, was surprisingly a period of rapid growth and development at the Medical Center. The world's first lung and heart transplants were in 1963 and 1964. The second heart and lung transplants came in 1969. Work on both the artificial heart and electrical anesthesia garnered national headlines. Construction boomed during the decade, also. The nurses' dorm, the men's dorm (later renovated for the School of Health Related Professions), additional student apartments, the research wing, the nursing school building, the south hospital wing, and the first children's hospital were all built during the 1960s.

The original round children's hospital and the south hospital wing for adults were completed in 1968, heralding the beginning of a new era in pediatric care for the state. For Blair Batson, the chairman of pediatrics, the round hospital was the culmination of many years of working for a separate facility. Though physically connected to the main adult hospital, the new hospital gave pediatric patients their own clinics with child-sized furniture, their own radiology department, and their own pharmacy. Pediatric patients had occupied 7West of the original hospital. Pediatricians in town who needed to admit a patient had forty beds available to them, twenty-eight for pediatric medicine and twelve for pediatric surgery. "It was never enough," Batson said. "We frequently found ourselves having to turn down patients who needed to be here just because there wasn't room. Almost from the very beginning, it was obvious that we needed a hospital just for children." Batson's idea for the round construction was consistent with the realities of the time. The small rooms fanned out from the circular nurses' station that was always busy. "Most parents couldn't stay with children if they had to be hospitalized for a long time. I wanted the children to be able to watch the activity of the nurses' station." In 1955, Mississippi was still a rural state whose citizens had limited access to health care. During the first few years, the most common childhood illnesses treated by Batson and his colleagues were tuberculosis, scurvy, diphtheria, tetanus, typhoid fever, measles, pneumonia, polio, and roundworm. In a few short years, most of these diseases would virtually disappear from the practice of medicine owing to better antibiotics, improvements in plumbing, vaccinations, and more attention to the water supply. In 1955, there were no pediatric intensive care units, no newborn intensive care. Premature babies often died, and leukemia patients were sent home the afternoon they were diagnosed. "There was nothing we could do for them," Batson said. By 1968, pediatrics was a changed specialty. The new hospital allowed Batson to recruit pediatric specialists so that the children's hospital was now prepared to treat the whole range of childhood illnesses and conditions and become a pediatric referral center for the entire state. Beginning then, it became the only hospital in the state where children could be treated for cancer, hemophilia, congenital heart defects, developmental disorders, cystic fibrosis, seizures, and epilepsy. As standards of care changed, the new round hospital soon became overcrowded and obsolete. The new children's hospital that bears Batson's name was opened in 1997—a state-of-the-art pediatric hospital that is a constant reminder of one man's dedication to the health and well-being of children.

The state's first artificial kidney unit, under the direction of Dr. John Bower, was opened at the Medical Center in 1966 funded by a three-year grant from the Bureau of State Services of the DHEW, which extended the grant for another year in 1969. The Orwellian task of deciding who should be given the life-saving treatment was the job of a special committee who made its recommendation based on how well treatment would restore a patient to his or her former vocation. The same year the grant was extended marked the acquisition of another grant from the Vocational Rehabilitation Division of the State Department of Education to establish an area at the Medical Center to train dialysis recipients to do the treatment themselves at home. When Congress authorized Social Security to pay for dialysis, all the ethical questions and access issues became irrelevant. Everyone who needed dialysis got it, in outpatient units around the state. Bower eventually developed the satellite centers into private facilities, independent of the Medical Center, although there was always a unit at the Medical Center for hospitalized patients.

The Mississippi Regional Medical Program began in 1966 under the coordination of Dr. Guy Campbell, clinical associate professor of medicine at the Medical Center and chief of the pulmonary disease section of the VA Hospital. The federal program, which Marston directed for NIH, was designed to put money into communities, under the control of the community, to help alleviate health problems caused by cancer, heart disease, and stroke.

As the 1960s ended, the Medical Center had emerged from a crucible of events, both terrifying and full of promise. The next two decades would prove that the crucible had produced something of rare value.

CHAPTER 6

Surgical Ascendancy

The historic lung and heart transplants of 1963 and 1964 were surprising only to those outside the confines of the University of Mississippi Medical Center. Those who knew Dr. James D. Hardy, the person who planned, directed, and carried out the operations, knew they were the culmination of years of work in the laboratory by Hardy and his colleagues and of Hardy's ambitious plan to put his "enterprise in Mississippi" on the world map.

Hardy, chairman of the Department of Surgery from 1955 until 1987, was the first clinical chair recruited by Dean David Pankratz in 1953 while Hardy was the director of surgical research at the University of Tennessee in Memphis.

The legacy of his thirty-two-year career as chairman is astonishing. He amassed a scholarly record that is rarely equaled. He wrote or edited twenty-three books including two autobiographies; he published nearly six hundred papers in medical journals. He served as president of every major surgical society in the world. His research into the transplantation of organs led him from the laboratory to the operating room in 1963 when he and his team transplanted the lung from one human into another and in 1964 when they transplanted a chimpanzee heart into a dying man. They were the first lung and heart transplants in the world, proving for the first time, that a transplanted lung would breathe and a transplanted heart would beat. He ascended the heights of his profession, and he took with him the fledgling institution he represented. But as much as he gave to the world, he is remembered by his students as a constant presence in the operating room, always there when they needed him, and a demanding but highly effective teacher. He trained the majority of the surgeons now practicing in Mississippi or trained the person who trained them.

Hardy's gentlemanly conduct, his intellectual curiosity and his strong work ethic had their roots deep in Alabama. He grew up in Newala, about thirty-five miles south of Birmingham, where his father owned a lime manufacturing plant. Hardy and his twin brother Julian, born in 1918, were the first children of Fred Henry Hardy and Julia Poynor Hardy, who were fifty and thirty-five when they married in 1917. Eighteen months after the birth of the twins, the Hardy's had another son, Taylor. But the Hardy household also consisted of four children of Fred Hardy's by a previous marriage. It was altogether a happy family according to James Hardy. "My mother had an absolute dedication to winning the love and respect of her stepchildren," and they reciprocated in kind. Although not wealthy by today's standards, the family was comfortably well-off. Their stability was threatened by the Great Depression when there was no construction, little water purification and, therefore, no widespread use for lime. The family's home and business were almost lost for nonpayment of taxes, but during the national recovery begun in President Franklin Roosevelt's administration, business picked up, and as Hardy recalled, "we finally dug out of the pit."

James and Julian went to school for the first three years in the front parlor of their home, taught by their mother who was a *summa cum laude* graduate of the University of Alabama and member of Phi Beta Kappa. She also held an advanced degree in Latin from Columbia University. They entered fourth grade at the local public school at the age of eight, no doubt years ahead of the other, older fourth graders. Hardy credits his mother for instilling an insatiable intellectual curiosity and his father for teaching him the value of work.

The twins finished high school and enrolled in the University of Alabama as pre-med students. They weren't fascinated with medicine; they just knew they did not want to run the lime business after witnessing what their father went through during the depression. James liked farming, but didn't like the dependence on the vagaries of weather. He also thought of teaching English. His decision to enter pre-med was a casual one, the result of two of his older friends who suggested it. Julian, he said, followed his lead. The Hardy parents supported their decision even though it was a costly investment. In 1935, at seventeen, the twins traveled by car with their parents to the University of Alabama in Tuscaloosa, sixty miles away over dirt roads.

Socially, the first year of college was a great success for James. He played many hands of bridge, joined a fraternity, and went to all the football games as a member of the band. Academically, it was—to him—a disaster and source of great embarrassment. Although he made high marks in English and German, he failed trigonometry, the first time he had ever made a failing grade in school. Instead of loosening his resolve to study medicine, which he had only half-heartedly endorsed before, the failure made him determined, not only to finish pre-med, but to succeed. The next three years were markedly different, with far more emphasis on academics than extracurricular activities. But for the failing grade in trig, Hardy says he probably would have made Phi Beta Kappa.

Julian, by now engaged to an Alabama girl, decided to stay in Tuscaloosa to attend the university's two-year medical school. James, however, said he wanted to take all four years at the same school and heeded the advice of a local medical family to apply to the University of Pennsylvania. Having learned his lesson about study discipline during his first year of college, James fared well academically in competition with students from all over the Northeast. Julian transferred from Alabama their junior year, the same year their father died at age seventy-four. James was tapped for membership in Alpha Omega Alpha, the medical honorary society, and was elected president. He also won the Undergraduate Medical Association Research Prize. The Hardy twins graduated from Penn together in 1942, five months after the Japanese had bombed Pearl Harbor, initiating America's entry into World War II.

In his year of rotating internship at Penn, he liked medicine best, and at the end of the year was one of two selected for residencies in internal medicine at Penn. As he recalled in his memoirs, he very much liked and respected the department chairman Dr. O. H. Perry Pepper. During medical school, Hardy had taken ROTC and spent the summer between his second and third year training at Carlisle Barracks near Harrisburg. He would be commissioned as a second lieutenant after medical school. But university officials had persuaded the War Department that Hardy's services as a resident in medicine were essential to the running of the University Hospital, so Hardy's active duty was deferred. In the spring of 1944, however, Pepper asked Hardy to meet with Dr. Robert Loeb of Columbia-Presbyterian Medical Center in New York, who had been charged with assembling a research team to find a way to control the ravages of malaria among the American troops in the South Pacific. Pepper asked Hardy and a fellow resident, Franklin Murphy, to consider the job. Hardy accepted, and Penn officials removed Hardy's name from the "essential" list. War Department officials, while approving Murphy's assignment with the malaria research team, had a different notion of how Hardy could best serve his country. They said Hardy had trained with ground forces, and that was where they assigned him. A month after his meeting with Loeb, Hardy was headed back to Carlisle Barracks to receive his orders, his residency in medicine on temporary hold.

It would turn out to be the last of his training in internal medicine, but the year had given him crucial experience in research. While seeing all the patients assigned to him, he had also completed two research projects that sealed his lifelong passion for research. One was to compare the effects of IV fluid on normal subjects with patients who were dehydrated. The IV fluids substantially increased the cardiac output in dehydrated patients. The second project was determined to answer the question: do patients with low levels of protein in the blood absorb amino acids at the normal rate? The latter he did entirely alone, running all the chemical analysis in the lab himself. "Research is never quite the same as when an investigator does every analysis and calculation himself. He knows his data cold, something that is deeply satisfying," he wrote. He also noted, "Research became a vital part of my professional life during my residency and was to remain so thereafter. I learned that it is not necessary to be a genius or have some primordial insight to do useful research. One simply has to work hard at it and intelligently as one would otherwise be doing with patients."

On his first permanent assignment as a first lieutenant at Stark General Hospital in Charleston, South Carolina, he met Louise "Weezie" Scott Sams, who would become his wife five years later. A recent graduate of Agnes Scott College, which her forebears had founded, she was in Charleston for the duration of the war. Her father had been transferred from Atlanta by the Atlantic Coast Line railroad. Hardy's entry in the journal he kept during his active duty in the military described her as "a most delightful girl. Brown eyes, brown hair, yellow summer frock, high heels."

From McGuire General Hospital in Richmond, Virginia, Hardy asked to be assigned overseas "before the war ends." He spent the remainder of the war and his military career with the Eighty-first Field Hospital. The experience was to decide his future. He discovered that internal medicine was not where he wanted to spend his professional life. "In the Eighty-first I had the feeling, in the presence of wounded men, that I was something less than a complete physician. I needed a field to which I could devote, with complete dedication and without mental reservations, whatever abilities I might have."

He wrote to Pepper and the other medical chiefs at Penn telling them not to hold his residency open; he had decided to apply for a spot in the surgery residency at Penn under the famous Dr. Isidor S. Ravdin. It was Ravdin, more than any other individual, whose example molded Hardy's professional behavior. Hardy never flinched in his praise for his mentor and role model. He was everything Hardy wanted to be. His other two chief influences during his surgery residency were Dr. Jonathan Rhoads, namesake of the famous *Rhoads Textbook of Surgery*, and Dr. Julian Johnson, a pioneer in the new field of thoracic surgery. Hardy called him the finest surgeon he ever worked with.

After completing general surgery training, he was asked to stay on to train in thoracic surgery under both Johnson and Rhoads. In his last year at Penn, 1950–1951, he received a Damon Runyon Fellowship that paid $5,000 per year. With that sum he would be able to complete his heavy water research. His goal was to determine the amount of water a human body contains. "Heavy water" had been discovered in the 1930s, and Hardy reasoned that, since the concentration of heavy water in normal water was known, if he could inject a known quantity of heavy water in a human body, he could determine the overall fluid volume by measuring the amount of dilution. Heavy water occurs naturally in water, but must be separated out. The Norwegians had perfected the complicated process of producing heavy water, used in harnessing nuclear power, and Hardy had obtained two 25-gram sealed tubes from Norway for his research.

His reputation as a clinician-scientist was assured. Jonathan Rhoads had advised him that he wouldn't be happy in a place where he couldn't pursue his research objectives, and that many schools would welcome his talents at both surgery and research. He also finished his first book his last year at Penn, *Surgery and the Endocrine System*, published by W. B. Saunders. Hardy was torn about leaving Penn, his academic home for thirteen years. And Ravdin wanted him to stay, but the young surgeon thought it might be years before he achieved a position of leadership because able surgeons were already waiting in the wings for top posts.

On his way back from Texas, where he interviewed with both Dr. Michael DeBakey and Dr. Carl Moyer, he stopped in Memphis at the suggestion of Rhoads, who was a friend of Dr. Harwell Wilson, the chairman of surgery at the University of Tennessee in Memphis. Hardy decided Memphis was where he would bring his family. By now Hardy had married the yellow-frocked brunette he had met in Charleston and they had the first of their four daughters, Louise. He took the post of director of surgical research at UT in 1951.

Hardy proved a master at getting his research funded. In fact, at one point, he got more money than he could reasonably use. When he realized he would not have the time to devote to the research that the grant funded, he returned the money, much to the dismay of the vice chancellor, Dr. Orin W. Hyman. He had ample opportunity to expand his surgery practice with the vast numbers and variety of surgical problems presented by the patients at the John Gaston Hospital. He also expanded his thoracic surgery expertise by doing two lung surgeries a week at the West Tennessee Tuberculosis Hospital. He and a colleague did the first heart mitral valve surgery in the Memphis area. As in all of Hardy's endeavors, he was successful in Memphis, but there were several factors that limited his satisfaction with the job. He was the first and only full-time faculty member in the Department of Surgery, all others being in private practice and dependent on a practice income. He said this distinction, not common at Penn, made him something of a socialist in the minds of some physicians who, as a group, were keenly conservative. It was an issue that would come up again in Jackson when physicians on the faculty of the new medical school would be almost always full-time university employees. Memphis also lacked the open discussion of surgical mistakes that characterized the department at Penn. The mortality and morbidity conference that Hardy instituted at the University of Mississippi Medical Center (an open discussion of deaths and complications on the surgery service) was designed to remind surgeons they were always accountable to someone. Hardy says criticism at Memphis was often muted because most of the surgeons were in private practice and they declined to openly criticize their peers.

Hardy's years in Memphis coincided with the planning of Mississippi's four-year medical school and teaching hospital that would be built 210 miles to the south. David Pankratz, the dean of the two-year medical school at the University of Mississippi in Oxford (later to become the dean and director of the Medical Center when it opened in 1955), and Dr. Harwell Wilson were close friends, and apparently Pankratz engaged his advice on how Wilson's new recruit might fare as chairman of surgery in the new school in Jackson. In 1953, Pankratz offered Hardy the job as chairman of surgery, and Hardy accepted. Wilson and Hyman agreed that he could keep his job in Memphis until the Medical Center was built in Jackson.

So in 1955, with Weezie and four young daughters in tow, Hardy moved to Jackson. He brought with him several key personnel who would work for him for the next decades of their lives. Dr. M. Don Turner had just married his lab technician, Anne Cole Bass, and they came with Hardy. Both stayed at the Medical Center until their retirements, Don Turner as a professor of surgery (research) and chairman of the medical school admissions committee. Dr. William Neely was one of Hardy's residents who came with him. He joined the faculty in surgery when he completed his residency and remained at the Medical Center until his death. He also brought photographer John H. Dickson, who photographed all of Hardy's procedures for his scientific papers and produced the instructional movies that Hardy showed to audiences around the world. Thelma Carter, another lab technician, accompanied Hardy from Memphis as did as Dr. Jorge Rodrigues, a surgeon trained in Mexico. Virginia Keith (then Ward) had just finished college with a degree in chemistry when she applied for a position in Hardy's office in Memphis. It was the first job and only job interview she ever had. She started working for Hardy in Memphis, moved to Jackson when he came, and retired after being at the Medical Center forty years. Hardy called her "a bulldog on spelling." As it turned out, while her services in the lab were important to Hardy, it was Keith's impeccable editing and proofreading that made her such an indispensable part of his team. Keith remembers her former boss with a great deal of affection and respect. "He was unfailingly polite. He never asked any member of his office staff to get his coffee or do personal things for him." Hardy also depended on Keith, a voracious reader and bibliophile, to do his library searches for him. "He never forgot anything he ever read, but sometimes he couldn't remember where he had read it. It was my job to find the source of something he remembered."

Dr. Watts Webb was an indispensable member of the transplant research team. He came to see Hardy very early in Hardy's tenure and wanted to work for him. He was doing lung surgery at the Tuberculosis Sanatorium in Magee at the time. "I had filled all my slots, so I told him he could do 20 percent here and still do 80 percent at the Sanatorium," Hardy said. "After I had a chance to see him operate, I asked him to give the San 20 and us 80." Webb left in 1963, to become chairman of cardiothoracic surgery at the University of Texas Southwestern in Dallas—just weeks before the first heart transplant.

With his core staff in place, Hardy began to recruit other faculty in surgery. He hired Dr. Orlando Andy for neurosurgery, Dr. Glance Bittenbinder in anesthesiology, Dr. Curtis Artz and Dr. Watts Webb in general surgery, and Dr. William F. Enneking in orthopedics. Dr. James Hendrix, a surgeon in private practice, ran the plastic surgery service. Dr. Sam Johnson, the young son-in-law of Dr. Henry Boswell, directed the ophthalmology service. Boswell was a key ally of Dean Pankratz in gaining support for the Medical Center as well as an important leader in Mississippi. Pankratz asked Hardy to give Johnson the ophthalmology service, which he ran on a part-time basis for several years before joining the faculty full-time. In 1955, Johnson had recently completed ophthalmology training at Tulane University, and Hardy, for once, agreed with Pankratz on the appointment.

Pankratz asked Hardy to interview several candidates for chairs of other clinical departments, and the two often diverged in their opinions. Hardy wanted chairs, like him, who were strong in research as well as clinical skills, believing that if a chairman doesn't do research and publish, neither will the faculty. He believed that "there are no great medical school departments that do not have effective research in progress."

Hardy brought research grants and staff from Memphis, so his labs at the Medical Center were up and running almost from the first day. He continued to excel at both receiving grants and publishing the results of the work funded by the grants. He was also busy on another book, his fourth, *Pathophysiology in Surgery*, that would come out in 1958.

With his young family suitably housed near the Medical Center, Hardy lost no time setting up the labs and organizing the teaching program in surgery for the new medical school. Hardy had won the battle of board certification or board qualification for surgeons who operated in University Hospital. All surgeons with admitting privileges were either board certified by the American Board of Surgery or board eligible—those who had finished residency training but had not yet taken board exams.

By 1955, at the age of thirty-seven, he was chairman of a department of surgery and the author or coauthor of sixty-four papers (forty-three of which he was the first author) in scientific journals. He was well on his way to leaving a giant footprint in the world of surgery. World War II had greatly advanced the field of surgery. By the middle of the 1950s, new techniques in vascular surgery, the development of the heart lung machine, and new suture materials had made open heart surgery possible. Hardy was keenly aware that organ transplantation was the next enormous leap in surgery, and he wanted to be on the front lines early. He and Dr. Watts Webb began to do organ transplants in animals by 1956. He continued to write papers about his research and encourage his residents and faculty to do likewise. They were so productive, the attention they received wasn't exactly positive.

The Surgical Forum of the American College of Surgeons (ACS) is held annually during the college's Clinical Congress. The forum, begun in 1941, was "born out of the great need for young men, engaged in research on surgical problems, to have an opportunity to bring their work before an audience of surgeons." In 1951, the papers presented at the Forum were published for the first time in a single volume. From that point, publication in the volume was a career-enhancing achievement and greatly coveted. In 1957, the first year Hardy and his team went to the Forum, they had twenty papers accepted—a feat that was not applauded, but censored. Dr. Isidor Ravdin, Hardy's chairman at Penn and his esteemed mentor, was on the Board of Regents of the ACS at the time of the Mississippi "invasion." He wrote Hardy that the regents were "concerned that several university organizations were not given a place on the program while other organizations were given many places. This, of course, should never occur. Duke and Northwestern, although they turned in a number of requests, did not have a single place on the program. I hope this will not occur in the future."

Hardy, typically, responded deftly, and it is hard to imagine him writing the letter with a straight face. "Thank you so much for your letter regarding the Forum problems. I myself was astonished that Duke and Northwestern did not have a paper on the program, and I am sure that such omissions will be prevented in the future. I am confident that the Board of Regents will hand down a fair and practicable solution."

The next year, Hardy's team, not thoroughly chastened, had nineteen papers accepted for publication. In subsequent years, the college passed a resolution that limited the number of papers by a single institution. It became known as "the

Mississippi Rule." Over the course of his career as chairman of the department, Hardy and his colleagues contributed a total of 120 papers to the forum. Long after Hardy was no longer the young upstart who threatened the traditions of the surgical establishment, the Committee on the Forum of Fundamental Surgical Problems came full circle in 1983 when it dedicated the Surgical Forum XXXIV to Hardy "whose career exemplifies the application of scientific principles in clinical surgery." The dedication read further, "Throughout his remarkably productive career he has developed and effectively used his extensive scientific background to solve difficult clinical problems. He has been highly effective at the bedside application of theoretical knowledge."

The Mississippi team's prominence in publishing reflected vigorous work in the laboratory on a number of problems related to transplantation. In the transplantation of kidneys, Hardy said he and his team simply followed the lead of other innovators who had successfully transplanted kidneys in the early 1950s. But Hardy's team did pioneer a procedure in which they moved a person's kidney to the pelvis. This development came about because it was common practice to remove one kidney (sacrifice it) if the ureter was injured. The ureter is the tube leading from the kidney to the bladder. Hardy decided there was no need to sacrifice a kidney if he could move it and sew the shortened ureter to the bladder.

The team also did what they thought was the first adrenal gland transplant in the world. They learned later that a similar procedure had been done in New Zealand earlier. It was certainly the first in the United States. To treat Cushing's disease, the team removed the two adrenal glands in the abdomen, then transplanted slices of the adrenal tissue into a muscle of the thigh, supplying enough hormone so that the patient did not have to stay on replacement steroids for life. Hardy discontinued adrenal transplants when it became known that virtually all cases of Cushing's were caused by a tumor.

Hardy's team even transplanted a uterus in a dog in 1963. His interest in the operation was piqued when a gynecologist asked him if he could do such an operation on a patient of his, a young woman who had previously had a hysterectomy and now wanted to bear children. Hardy told him that he wouldn't even consider doing it in a human but he tried the procedure in dogs with considerable success. Two of the dogs not only survived, but had several litters. He concluded that if the immunology of rejection could be overcome, uterine transplants might be a viable treatment in some patients.

Between 1956 and 1963 Hardy, along with Dr. Watts Webb, Dr. Martin Dalton, and Dr. Fikri Alican, performed about one thousand lung transplants in animals.

He explained this phase of his career and the thoughts behind it to Jurgen Thorwald in *The Patients*, a book about the patients who volunteered for historic surgical procedures and thereby advanced the field of medicine. In the first stages of the research, to avoid the problem of rejection, they perfected surgical techniques simply by removing a lung from the animal and then re-implanting the same lung in the same animal. Later they moved to transplanting the lung from one animal into another animal's chest. They discovered that they had to leave behind a part of the old lung so that the new lung would be connected to the same respiration centers in the brain. And they discovered that a lung had to be continuously supplied with oxygen until it had been sewn into the recipient's bronchial stem. Hardy said the lungs would function in the animals for seven days until the body rejected it. By 1961 or 1962, transplant scientists began reporting on results with Imuran, the first truly effective anti-rejection, or immunosuppressive, drug. Of thirty-four dogs in Hardy's lab with transplanted lungs, twenty lived thirty days with Imuran.

With the possibility of a transplanted lung lasting several weeks, Hardy said he told his team he wanted to move from animals to humans. He wanted to do a human transplant and got permission from Dr. Robert Marston, the dean and Medical Center director. Hardy had seen several cases in the previous months in which a lung transplant, though experimental, would be morally acceptable and clinically useful. Patients who vomited the contents of their stomachs while unconscious and sucked the contents into their lungs often died before the lungs had a chance to heal. The acid from the stomach contents paralyzes the lungs, but if the patient can live long enough, it will eventually heal. A transplanted lung, even if it lasted only a few weeks, would take over the respiration for one damaged lung while it healed. Even when the new lung was rejected, the patient would be left with one healthy lung.

In seeking institutional approval for the world's first human lung transplant, Hardy gave Marston these assurances: (1) The recipient of the new lung would almost certainly have a fatal disease. If the operation went sour, it could not be argued that the transplant shortened his life. (2) There must be a "reasonable possibility" that the patient would benefit from the transplant. (3) Removal of the patient's diseased lung would not result in the sacrifice of a significant amount of the patient's own functioning lung tissue. (4) The lung to be replaced would be the left lung because it has longer, unbranched portions of the pulmonary artery and main bronchus and was technically easier than the right lung. Therefore, Hardy met today's ethical requirements for an experimental procedure before they were ever conceived. He had presented a pre-determined set of guidelines and waited for the patient who would meet them.

The donor requirements were much more stringent than they would be today because the classification of death by the cessation of brain activity did not exist. Death was determined only after the heart stopped beating and the lungs stopped breathing.

On April 15, 1963, the patient who would make medical history was admitted to University Hospital. He was John Russell, a prisoner at Parchman, the state penitentiary. At fifty-eight, he had been an inmate for the past six years serving a life sentence for the murder of a fourteen-year-old boy. Russell had confessed to the killing immediately after it happened. Witnesses said Russell, known to be a binge drinker on the weekends, went to the home of a woman he liked and found a noisy group of poker players on her porch. He began firing his pistol wildly, and the boy got hit as the other men scattered. It was a desperately irresponsible act, but not murder in the usual sense. Even the sheriff who arrested Russell was surprised at the court's verdict.

For several months before his admission, Russell had been given antibiotics for six or seven bouts of pneumonia. The drugs didn't help, and Russell's breathing became more and more difficult. The slightest activity brought on spasms of coughing and bloody mucous. At the hospital, where Medical Center physicians routinely treated prisoners referred by prison doctors, Russell's chest x-ray and lung biopsy revealed cancer of the left lung. He had about a third of the lung capacity of healthy people. He fought for every breath, and when he was told he had cancer and the lung should be removed, his only question was, "Will I be able to breathe a little easier?" He also had kidney disease, which would inevitably lead to renal failure. Hardy was convinced that Russell was the patient who met the guidelines he had proposed. If his left lung, where the squamous cell tumor was located, were removed, he would likely die within weeks from the spread of cancer or the kidney failure. And the right lung, so compromised from emphysema, probably could not handle total respiration. When Hardy talked to Russell about volunteering for the transplant, neither he nor Russell mentioned a possible pardon in exchange for volunteering for an experimental surgery. By not making promises about a commutation in sentencing, Hardy was abiding by later ethical guidelines that condemned coercion of experimental subjects. After deliberating several days and talking with his family, Russell decided to have the transplant.

On June 11, almost two months after Russell had been admitted to the hospital, a donor lung became available. Martin Dalton was the senior thoracic surgery resident at the time and immediately recognized that the patient who had died of a massive heart attack would have a lung suitable for transplant. The family consented, and the transplant was underway.

Dr. Mart McMullan, a Jackson heart surgeon, was a medical student at the time of the transplant. He had been working in Hardy's research lab during the summer so he knew of the plans for the operation. "I watched as the nurse anesthetist ventilated the donor lung. It just looked so funny to me. She asked me if I wanted to do it." McMullan was a third-year resident by the time Hardy did the second lung transplant in 1969.

The major problem the surgeons encountered in 1963 was the size of the donor lung compared to the shrunken chest cavity of the recipient. They thought the whole operation might be in jeopardy, but Hardy kept pushing the lung into the space and finally made it fit. When the final sutures were made, Hardy prepared to close. With about an hour left to finish, the OR team got an urgent call to report to the emergency room.

Dalton, whose main job was in retrieving the donor organ, had finished his most important work, so Hardy asked Dalton to go to the ER while he closed. Dalton flew down the stairs to find a young black man with a gunshot wound. He had been shot at close range with a rifle. The entry wound was small, but the exit wound was "massive." The chest was opened, and Dalton attempted to stop the bleeding. He used manual heart massage and defibrillation—all to no avail. Thirty minutes later, Dalton pronounced death, still not knowing the identity of the man he tried to save. Only after he told those gathered in the waiting room the sad news, was he informed that the man was Medgar Evers, the civil rights activist who had been shot on his front porch by radical white supremacists.

Leaving the operating room, Hardy and the others well understood the significance of their achievement. They were the first to remove a human lung and replace it with the lung from another person. They discovered that the noise and heightened level of activity outside the OR that night was not about their history-making operation but about the murder of Medgar Evers. It was one of those examples of the parallel universe Mississippians inhabited in that era—a signal achievement that represented the best impulses of humankind happening almost simultaneously with an act of cowardice and evil from humanity's dark underside. For Dalton, who recounted the experience in 1995, it "was one of the most bittersweet days of my life." He had played a major role in the lung transplant and in the efforts to save the life of a hero.

The next day, while Russell was still breathing with mechanical support, the news of the transplant barely caused a ripple in the national media. Jackson's local newspaper, the *Clarion-Ledger*, ran the story below the fold; the Evers assassination was the lead story. Hardy never spoke to reporters, always deferring to Maurine

Twiss, the Medical Center's director of public relations. For that he gets praise from Mary Jo Festle in her 2002 examination of the operation and its aftermath in the *Journal of Mississippi History*. She specifically looked at the operation in light of subsequent ethical guidelines for experimental procedures in humans and judged Hardy's conduct both professional and ethical. Of course, the Medical Center's public relations office was still operating under the Central Medical Society's guidelines for "physician advertising" that forbade the use of a physician's name in connection with news of a new clinical treatment no matter how significant the advance.

The patient in this landmark surgical case was indifferent to such considerations. The day the story appeared in the newspaper was day one of Russell's new lung—and it was working. Tests indicated to Hardy that the lung was suffused with blood, and he decided to take Russell off mechanical support. Russell got what he wanted most in his world of lowered expectations—improved breathing. Dalton said his oxygen saturation post transplant was seven times what it was before the surgery. He lived eighteen days after the operation. Ironically, when Russell died, his new lung was still working and showing no signs of rejection. But Russell's kidneys stopped functioning entirely, and he died of renal failure on June 29. Hardy said hemodialysis could have saved his patient, or at least significantly prolonged his life. Artificial kidney units, in which the blood from the patient is filtered through a machine and returned the patient, were not widely available in 1963, and University Hospital did not have one. Hardy had to rely on peritoneal dialysis, which was not effective in taking over the function of Russell's failing kidneys.

The patient's death notwithstanding, the operation in Hardy's view was a success. The lung worked. It got the signals from the brain to breathe even though it was from another person's body. It saturated the body with oxygen. And if the lung, why not the heart? Dr. Watts Webb had begun the animal heart transplant program in 1956, and he and Hardy had published several papers. Now Hardy began his preparations for taking the work from animals to humans. He again talked with Marston and got approval to proceed with a heart transplant if the criteria for both donor and recipient, already outlined, could be met. In the animal labs, Hardy organized donor and recipient teams, and each rehearsed the transplant many times in animals. The donor team opened the chest of the donor, removed the heart, and quickly cooled it in an iced salt solution. The other team connected the recipient to the heart-lung machine, opened the chest, and took out the old heart.

Interestingly, part of Hardy's preparation was taking the pulse of the professional and lay community. In many settings, both among colleagues and in social groups, he tested the waters of public opinion on the issue of heart transplantation. He knew, going in, what a firestorm he was about to create.

In the weeks and months before the heart transplant, it seemed unlikely that a patient destined to be donor would die at precisely the same time that a recipient needed a heart. All measures, of course, had to be attempted to save a dying heart and the failing heart had to stop beating before donation could be considered. There was no brain death classification. Fearing that such a confluence of circumstances would never come about, Hardy bought four large chimpanzees based on the work of Dr. Keith Reemtsma, a Hardy trainee, at Tulane University. Hardy was impressed because Reemtsma had transplanted a kidney from a chimp into a person who was doing well post transplant. The chimps, man's closest genetic relative, would be held in reserve if they were needed. Hardy knew he was in for adverse reactions now. If the idea of heart transplants was alien to people, how would the world react to a chimp heart in a man?

With Marston alerted, both donor and recipient teams rehearsed and ready, and chimpanzees waiting in the wings if a human donor weren't available, Hardy and his colleagues watched for patients who might meet the criteria for a transplant. They thought the man who came in on January 11 was that person. The patient was referred by one of Hardy's former students in Laurel, ninety miles to the south of Jackson. The patient's heart, injured by a stab wound, was now throwing clots. Clots had blocked an artery to the brain, leaving the patient mentally confused and partially paralyzed; others had blocked arteries to both legs resulting in amputations; and another had blocked an intestinal artery. Dr. Sam Robinson, Hardy's former student, thought the patient's only chance of survival was to remove the injured, clot-making heart. Hardy thought so, too, until he saw the patient.

For all of those who criticized Hardy for moving too fast, blind to the needs of the patients in these experimental procedures, this patient was proof of Hardy's clinical integrity. As it turned out, Hardy was able to repair the patient's heart and to stop the disabling production of clots—at the same time a suitable human donor heart was available.

The operation on January 18 served as a practice run that convinced Hardy's team they were ready to replace a human heart. That opportunity came when Robinson called Hardy about another patient in his hospital—Boyd Rush. Rush was a deaf mute who lived alone in a trailer in Hattiesburg, Mississippi. He was retired from his job as an upholsterer, and his wife was dead. He had moved to Hattiesburg to be near a church where deaf people worshiped and formed a close community.

Affable and friendly, he worked as a peddler selling pots and pans door-to-door. His neighbor had alerted authorities when she noticed that Rush had not left his trailer, yet his car was in the driveway and she couldn't get him to the door. They found him on the floor unconscious. He had apparently fallen from a chair while changing a light bulb. From the time of his apparent fall on January 20 until the transplant on January 23, he never regained consciousness.

Robinson, the same surgeon who had sent the first patient to Hardy, thought Rush might meet Hardy's criteria as the recipient of a heart. By the time Rush got to Jackson, he was in a rapid decline. The cardiologist who examined him said he would probably be dead within hours. Hardy talked to Rush's only known relative, a stepsister who had come from Cleveland, Mississippi, to be with her brother. She gave permission for a heart transplant with the understanding that it would be the first heart transplant in a human and that the heart itself might be a chimpanzee heart.

When Hardy got word that a patient with a severe brain injury was in the intensive care unit and not expected to live, Hardy got his teams ready. The patient was breathing only with mechanical support; his brain was not functioning. But no one knew when the heart would stop. Hardy was trying to keep Rush alive until the donor's heart stopped beating, but Rush's blood pressure dropped, and he was going into shock. They had to give him large quantities of drugs to maintain his blood pressure. Hardy regularly sent one of his team to the intensive care unit to monitor the donor. Every report had the donor's heart still beating vigorously. Rush was near death, so Hardy ordered the donor team to retrieve the heart of the largest chimpanzee. Hardy and his team knew that the transplant would not save Rush's life. It might, however, give him a few hours or days of conscious awareness.

As Dr. William Turner, the James D. Hardy Professor of Surgery at the Medical Center and chair of the Department of Surgery, put it more than three decades later, James D. Hardy was the first person to look inside the empty chest cavity of a human being and certainly the first to sew a replacement heart inside that cavity. Hardy himself called the empty chest "an awesome sight." Technically, the operation held no surprises. In fact, it was somewhat easier than the animal surgeries. The vessels of his human patient were larger and easier to work with than the vessels of the dogs he used in the laboratory. The heart began to beat as soon as Hardy removed the clamps from the vessels, and the electrical defibrillator produced a normal rhythm. For ninety minutes the heart sustained Rush's blood pressure, but the beat gradually weakened and faltered.

In the immediate aftermath of the transplant, the news traveled around the world. Letters from heart patients or their family members from all over the world flooded the post office at the Medical Center. The writers took the news of the heart transplant as a beacon of hope in their struggle for life. The medical community was not as enthusiastic. Hardy's first indication of the reaction came two weeks later when he was asked to participate in a panel discussion at the Sixth International Transplantation Conference in New York. Reemtsma, Hardy's former resident and transplant researcher at Tulane, spoke about his human kidney transplants using chimpanzee kidneys. The moderator, Willem Kolff, the inventor of the artificial kidney unit, called Hardy's name, but before Hardy could speak, Kolff said to the large audience, "In Mississippi, they keep the chimpanzees in one cage and the Negroes in another cage, don't they, Dr. Hardy?" With that one question, Hardy confronted Mississippi's contorted image to the rest of the world, and that view was affecting how people saw his work. Hardy had no sympathy for the white supremacist groups responsible for the violence against civil rights leaders in Mississippi. He was appalled by their actions as many Mississippians were. And he was appalled that anyone would think any notion of race would affect his work at all. His patients had been chosen very carefully on the basis of their physical condition, not their race. Russell was white; the man first considered for a heart transplant, but whose heart Hardy repaired instead of replaced, was black. Rush was also white.

Hardy says he was "taken aback" and fumbled through his presentation, one of the few times, he writes, that he "did poorly." He ended his account of the heart transplant to silence. Not a single person in the room applauded. According to Hardy, the California transplant pioneer, Dr. Norman Shumway, who followed Hardy on the panel, said some "positive things" about Hardy's operation, but on the whole, "it was a dismal day." About the same time, the Society of University Surgeons, of which Hardy was a past president, rescinded its decision to have its annual meeting in Jackson. Hardy never knew whether the decision was based on the racial turmoil in Mississippi or the negative reaction to the heart transplant. Hardy describes the aftermath of the heart transplant as a "searing" experience. "It was the first time my clinical integrity had ever been challenged. It hardened me forever . . ."

Criticism from his peers softened when his paper appeared in the *Journal of the American Medical Association* in June 1964. The paper detailed the strict guidelines Hardy and his team used in selecting both the donor and the recipient. And Hardy found, much to his delight, that European scientists and clinicians, unlike his American peers, were enthusiastic in their support of his pioneering surgery and wanted to know when he would do another.

But nationally and in Jackson, transplantation was quelled. Granting agencies were taking a long look at research in humans, and no group wanted to risk losing grant funds until guidelines were clear. Transplantation efforts had not been successful, due largely to the problem of rejection. And in 1964, agencies were still reeling from the scandal at the Jewish Chronic Disease Hospital in Brooklyn, New York, where researchers, in July of 1963, had injected cancer cells into patients who did not have cancer. Thus the inclination among scientists doing clinical research in 1964 was to turn their attention back to the animal labs.

The 1967 announcement that Christiaan Barnard had performed a heart transplant in South Africa shocked everyone, especially a transplant community that knew Barnard had done little research in the area. It shocked Hardy because he thought Shumway's group at Stanford would almost certainly be the next to do a heart transplant. They had vast experience in the lab and were well published, and it was Shumway's techniques that Hardy had used in the Boyd Rush transplant. It also ignited the government funding agencies that did not want the United States left behind in the new surgical frontier. Two weeks after the announcement the government's granting agencies, in an almost overnight change of heart, called him and other transplant surgeons to a meeting at O'Hare Airport in Chicago to plan for the future of transplantation in America.

Still, it would be 1969 before the Hardy team transplanted a heart and lung. On January 6, 1969, Russell Whitten of Marks, Mississippi, dying of heart disease, received a human heart—not beating, but preserved with a cold solution. He died within twenty-four hours from a blood vessel that burst in his brain. Frank McCurley, who received a human lung on January 18, fared better. He had come into the hospital unconscious and exhausted from severe emphysema in both lungs. He lived almost four weeks. On solid foods and off the respirator, he was scheduled to leave the hospital the day he developed an infection in the lungs. He had received the immunosuppressive drugs then available, and no rejection was evident at autopsy.

Hardy never said why these were the last transplants he attempted. He does not mention them in either of his two autobiographies. He does say that the early 1970s were marked by hostility from faculty from other departments who told him quite openly they wanted him gone. He may have thought he needed a lower profile to survive the threat. The resignation of Dr. Leonard Fabian as chair of anesthesiology made anesthesiology support tenuous until another chairperson could be recruited. He also recognized two major hurdles that had to be overcome before transplantation could ever be a viable clinical treatment. As long as a person wasn't declared dead until the heart stopped beating, donor hearts would not be in optimum health at transplant. Transplantation didn't really become effective until the courts ruled that a person could be declared dead when his brain stopped functioning. In that case, the heart could be removed while it was still beating. Truly effective drugs to allow the body to accept an organ from another person weren't available until the 1980s when Dr. Seshadri Raju reinstated the transplant program at the Medical Center.

By the early 1970s, Hardy began to assume a major role in national and international surgery circles. In 1970 he was appointed to the American Board of Surgery, the body that determines the content of exams given to surgeons seeking certification. From 1969 until 1973 he was a member of the American College of Surgeons' program committee and chair of the college's Committee on Pre- and Postoperative Care. By 1980, he had moved up through the college ranks and was elected president. In 1972, he was president of the Southern Surgical Association, and in 1975, he was elected president of the American Surgical Association. He was president of the Society of Surgical Chairmen from 1976 through 1978. In 1985, he was installed as president of the International Society of Surgery at its meeting in Paris. After the lung transplant in 1963 and the heart in 1964, he was increasingly in demand on the visiting professor circuit. In 1969 alone, he accepted invitations to lecture at the University of Pennsylvania, the University of Aberdeen in Scotland, New York University, the University of Kentucky, and Baylor Medical Center in Dallas.

Hardy did not stop writing papers and submitting them for publication. By 1970, he had written or edited twelve books and 350 papers. Dr. Mart McMullan, a resident of Hardy's during this time and a founding member of the Hardy Society, described what it was like to be a part of the Hardy team during this period of intense scholarly and clinical activity. "I really don't know when he slept," McMullan said. "He seemed to squeeze thirty-six hours into twenty-four. We often called him in the middle of the night because he always wanted to know what was going on with patients. And often, when we did, he'd be awake, writing. He never failed to be at the hospital in time for early rounds, and sometimes he'd leave rounds and go to the airport for a flight out. He seemed never to tire. He was indefatigable, a word he taught me, by the way. He also never came to the hospital, even to the emergency room in the middle of the night, dressed in anything but a coat and tie. He lived by a set of rules and manners that doesn't exist today. Going to national surgery meetings was exciting for us because everyone knew Dr. Hardy. And we were his boys." When McMullan went to the esteemed Mayo Clinic in Rochester, Minnesota, for a residency in cardio-thoracic surgery, "everyone knew who Dr. Hardy was, and I was respected because they all knew I had trained under Dr. Hardy."

Politically, the entire decade of the 1970s was a difficult time for the surgery chair. Hardy struggled with what he called "restive" divisions in the Department of

The University of Mississippi Medical Center

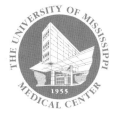

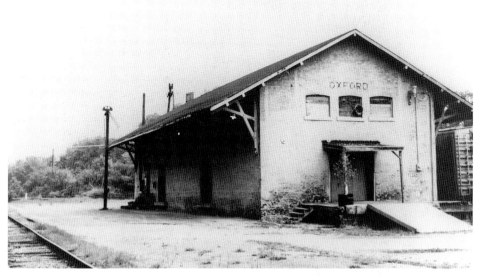

The Oxford depot as it was when Dr. Billy Guyton traveled by train in the course of his duties as dean of the medical school. One overnight trip to Jackson in 1936, for which Guyton submitted an expense summary to the university chancellor Alfred Butts, cost $5.24, including one meal on the train, three in Jackson, one night in a hotel, and taxi fare. Guyton tells Butts, "I used my railroad pass for transportation." Photo courtesy of the Mississippi Department of Archives and History.

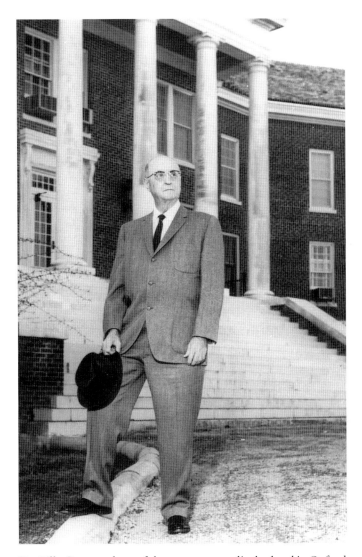

Dr. Billy Guyton, dean of the two-year medical school in Oxford from 1935 until 1944, stands in front of the medical school building named for him in 1961. Guyton saved the accreditation of the school, thereby assuring the successful establishment of the four-year school and teaching hospital in Jackson.

State Representative Zelma Price came to the state capitol in 1950 from her hospital bed to vote for the legislation that established the University of Mississippi Medical Center in Jackson.

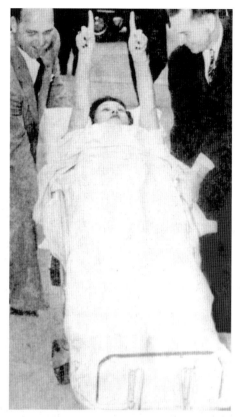

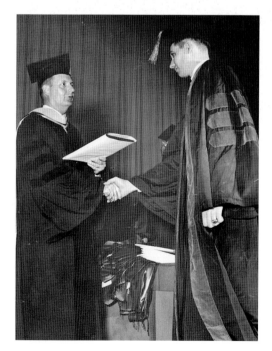

University chancellor J. D. Williams, left, presents the first four-year medical degree in Mississippi to Charles "Catfish" Allen during the Medical Center's first commencement ceremony in 1957.

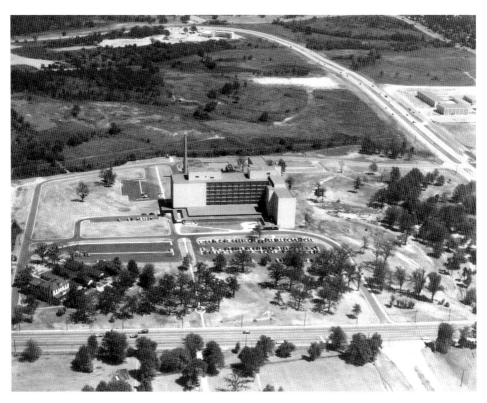

The "T" of the original Medical Center in 1955 is barely discernible in 2005 as the complex has grown up and around the nucleus. The original 491,498 square feet made it the biggest building in Mississippi in 1955.

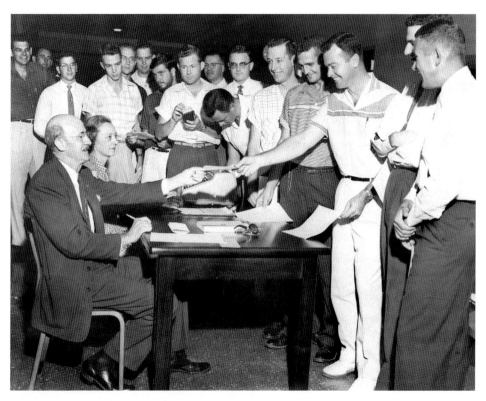

Dean David S. Pankratz, left, personally registered the first medical and graduate students in 1955 with the assistance of registrar Lallah Mayfield White, seated to his left.

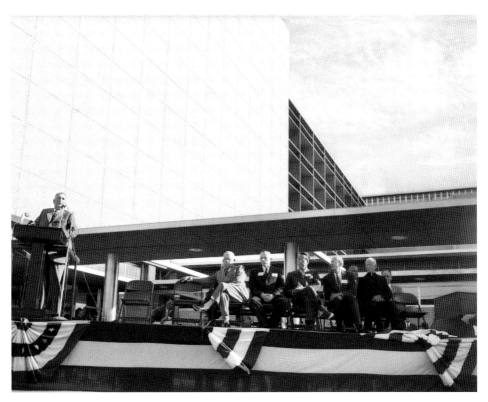

The public dedication of the Medical Center in October 1955 attracted four thousand Mississippians who came to tour the brand-new building.

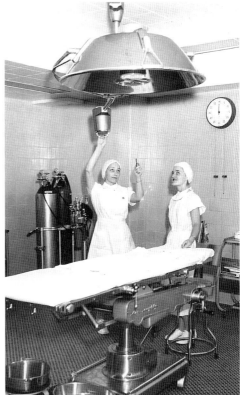

During public tours of the new building in 1955, Imogene Penn, operating room head nurse, demonstrated equipment in one of the new surgical suites.

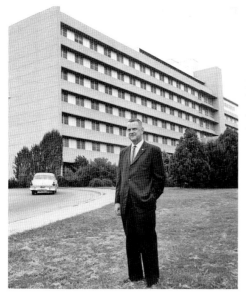

Dr. David Wilson, the first director of University Hospital, had the monumental task of getting the hospital up and running by the opening date, July 1, 1955.

Maurine Twiss, the Medical Center's first director of public information, was hired in 1955. A big part of her job was telling the state-at-large about the new Medical Center they paid for. In doing so, she fell into the center of the early controversy over physician "advertisement" with some local medical groups.

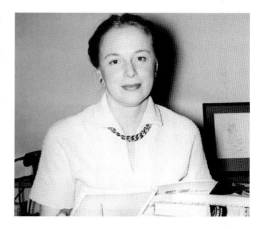

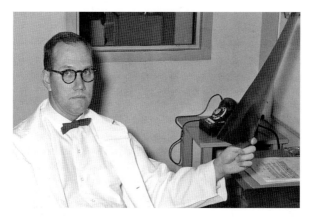

Dr. Robert Sloan, the first chair of radiology, held the post until he retired. He was also the first chair of the committee on minority recruitment in 1971.

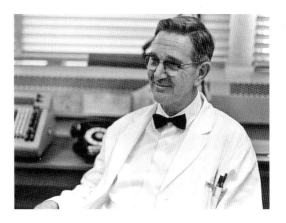

Dr. Thomas Brooks was the first chair of preventive medicine. Brooks helped plan the building for the four-year school when he was teaching at Oxford.

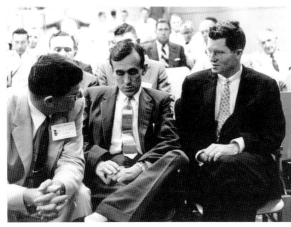

Dr. James D. Hardy, right, during an early continuing education course for physicians attended by Dr. Manning Hudson, center, a Jackson internist who served on the clinical faculty.

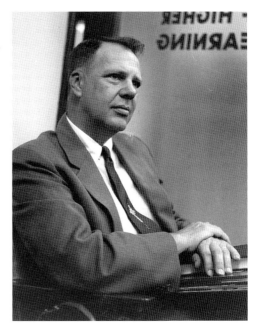

Frank Zimmerman, the Medical Center's first financial officer, served under Deans Pankratz, Marston, Carter, Blount, and Nelson.

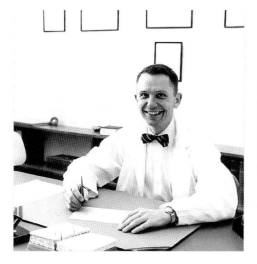

Dr. Thomas M. "Peter" Blake was appointed to the faculty in the Department of Medicine in 1955. He was a favorite of medical students until his death in 2002. He continued to interpret EKGs for cardiology long after his retirement.

Young Dr. Arthur C. Guyton was chair of physiology at the two-year school, then moved with the school when it came to Jackson as the first chair of physiology and biophysics. He retired as chair in 1987 but continued to teach and work on his textbook until he died in an automobile accident in 2003.

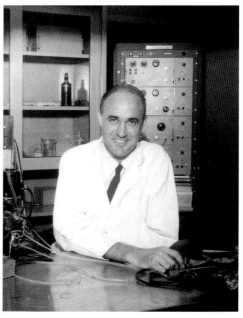

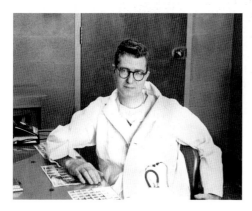

Dr. James D. Hardy was one of the youngest chairs of a department of surgery in the country at the time the Medical Center opened in 1955. His insistence that only board-certified surgeons could admit patients to the surgical service put him at odds with the local surgeons, many of whom were not board certified.

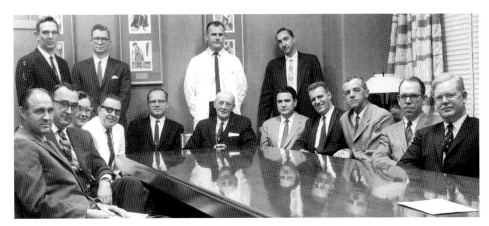

Dr. David S. Pankratz, seated center, resigned as dean in 1961 rather than face mandatory retirement. He left to enter a psychiatry residency at the University of Tennessee. His final meeting with the department chairs (members of the executive faculty) included, seated from left, Arthur Guyton, physiology; Foy Jack "Flick" Moore, psychiatry; Lucy Lawson (representing Charles Randall, chair of microbiology); Lane Williams, anatomy; Louis Sulya, biochemistry; standing from left, Thomas Brooks, preventive medicine; James Hardy, surgery; standing center (behind Pankratz), Joel Brunson, pathology; and seated from right, Mike Newton, ob-gyn; Blair Batson, pediatrics; Robert Snavely, medicine; Warren Bell, clinical labs; Julian Youmans (representing Orlando Andy, neurosurgery); and standing behind Youmans, Leonard Fabian, anesthesiology.

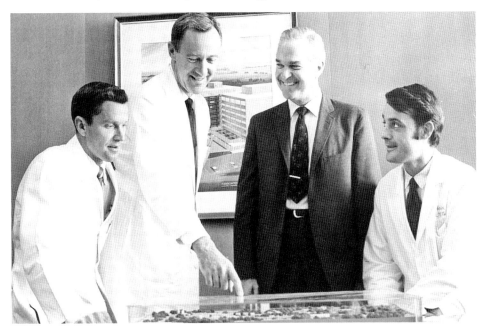

Robert Q. Marston, standing right, was appointed dean and Medical Center director after Pankratz resigned. He stayed until 1966 when he was tapped by the National Institutes of Health as associate director to head the Regional Medical Programs. He was succeeded by Dr. Robert E. Carter, standing left, who was dean until 1970. Marston, who maintained ties with the Medical Center long after he left, was back in Jackson for a visit, and Carter got him up to date on the progress of the long-range plan.

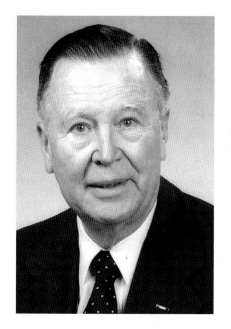

Dr. Robert E. Blount served as dean and Medical Center director after Carter resigned, from 1970 until Norman Nelson was appointed in 1973.

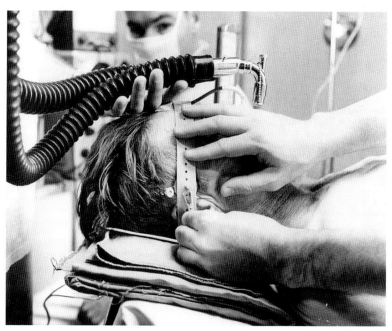

Dr. Leonard Fabian, chair of anesthesiology, pioneered electrical anesthesia at the Medical Center and received national acclaim, but better drugs eliminated the need for the procedure.

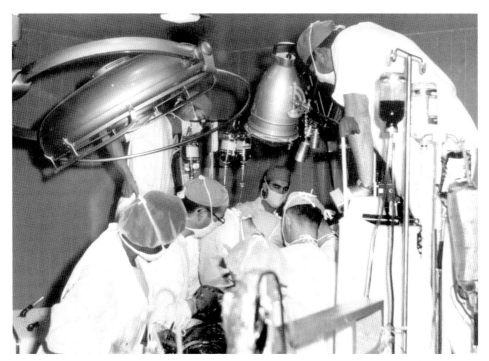
A scene in the operating room as Dr. James D. Hardy transplanted a chimpanzee heart in the body of Boyd Rush, who was dying of heart failure.

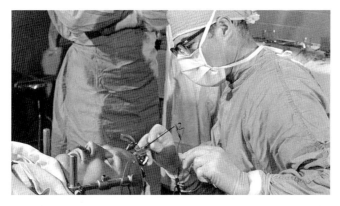

Dr. Orlando Andy, a member of the original faculty and later chair of neurosurgery, pioneered "psychosurgery," for which he was reviled in some quarters, hailed in others. His critics have been silenced as his techniques proved both safe and effective.

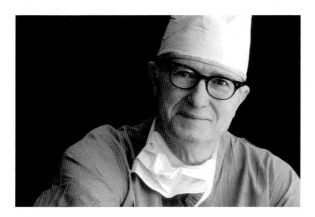

Dr. James Hardy as photographed by Communication Arts for the Mississippi exhibit at the World's Fair in New Orleans.

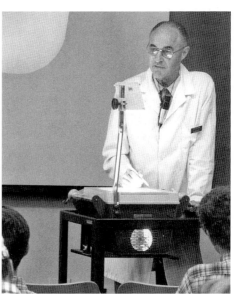

Dr. Arthur C. Guyton in his typical teaching position. Although dependent on crutches, he refused to teach from his wheelchair. He preferred standing so he could draw on the overhead projector.

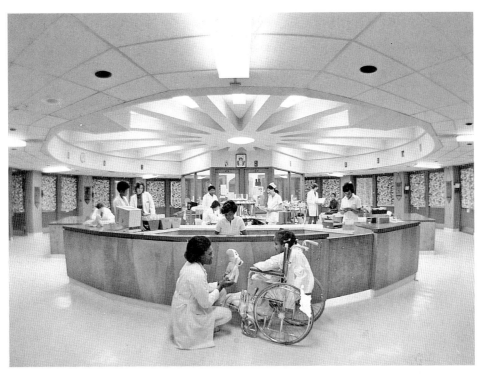

The original round children's hospital when it was new in 1968. Rooms opened up to the nurses' station so children could watch the activity.

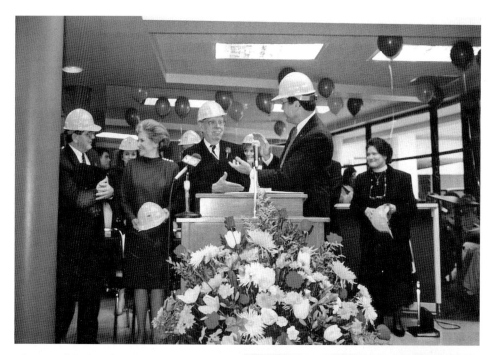

The 1995 "sky breaking" for the new Blair E. Batson Hospital for Children recognized the many contributions to the health of children by Dr. Blair E. Batson, center. The new children's hospital was built on top of the Mississippi Children's Cancer Clinic, so a traditional ground-breaking wasn't possible.

Will Searcy, a medical student, talks to a class of high school students in the program sponsored by the Medical Center chapter of Doctors Ought to Care (DOC). Searcy entered the family medicine residency at the Medical Center and was in the first group to complete it in 1976.

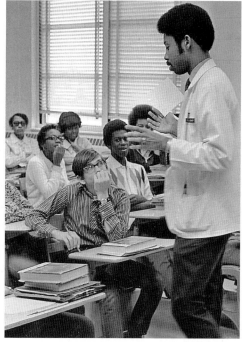

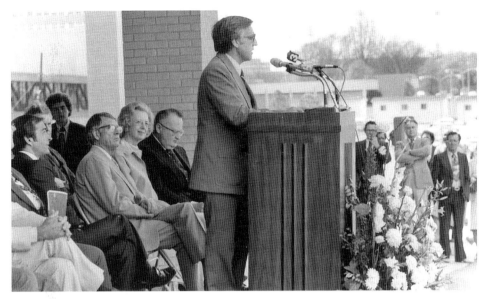

Dr. Wallace Mann, first dean of the dental school, speaks at the formal dedication of the new building for the school in 1977.

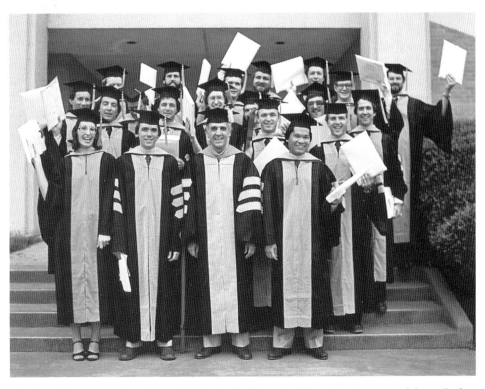

The first class to graduate from Mississippi's School of Dentistry in 1979 celebrated after the ceremony.

The orthodontic research project in the brand-new School of Dentistry that studied the movement of hamster teeth attracted national attention after this photo of the hamster in braces appeared in 1977.

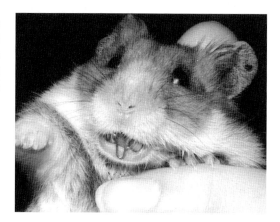

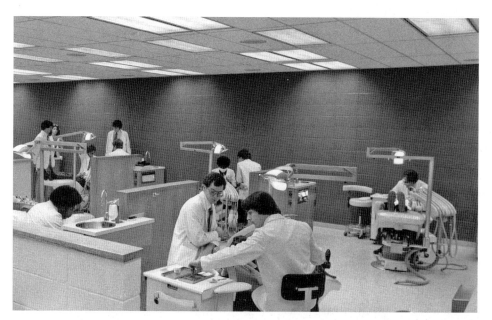

The School of Dentistry building, completed in 1977, still receives high marks from accrediting bodies for its efficient design and open operatories.

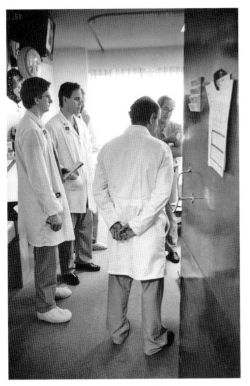

Dr. Bobby Heath, the heart surgeon, conducts rounds with students and residents. He was the state's only pediatric heart surgeon for many years and operated on hundreds of patients to correct congenital heart defects. Heath died in a diving accident in 2000.

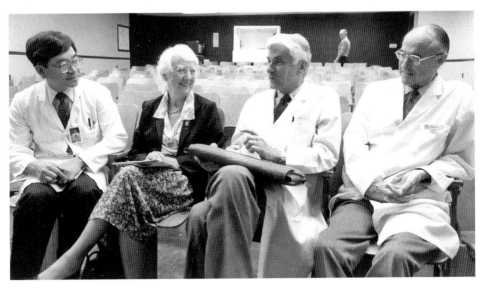

Dr. I. K. Ho, left, chair of pharmacology and toxicology, welcomed Dr. Harriet Duston, center left, as a guest lecturer in 1986. Dr. Herbert Langford, center right, and Dr. Arthur Guyton, right, talked to her about her work as director of the Cardiovascular Training Research Center at the University of Alabama before the lecture. Ho, still chair of pharmacology and toxicology, is also now dean of the School of Graduate Studies in the Health Sciences.

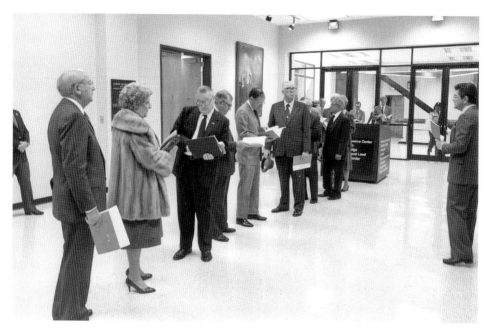

The dedication of the Verner S. Holmes Learning Resources Center honored Dr. Holmes, left, for his twenty-four-year tenure on the IHL board and for his support of the Medical Center all of his professional life. Other program participants getting ready for the 1983 dedication included Mrs. Holmes, Dr. Norman C. Nelson, Chancellor Porter Fortune, and Governors William Winter and J. P. Coleman.

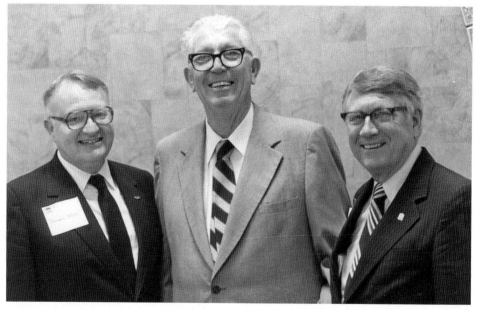

Governor James P. Coleman, center, was a great friend to the Medical Center as well as a patient on several occasions. He was always greeted warmly by Dr. Norman Nelson, left, and Chancellor Porter Fortune, right.

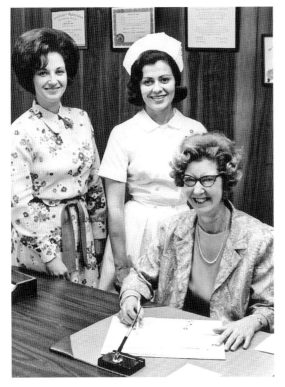

On School of Nursing Day in 1970, school dean Christine Oglevee, seated, posed with Edrie George, center, and Betty Preston. Preston was president of the Nursing Alumni Chapter in 1967 and was Alumni of the Year in 1971. George was Alumni of the Year in 1972 and succeeded Oglevee as dean when she retired.

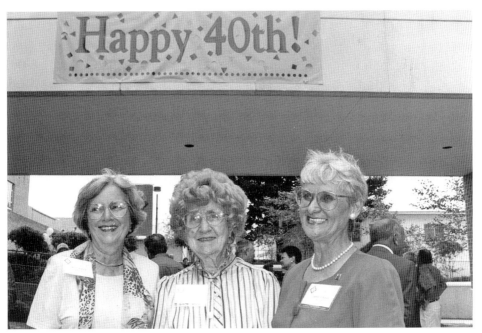

Mary Howard, Laura Blair, and Martha Bercaw, left to right, nursing school graduates in the Medical Center's first commencement of 1957, got together at the Medical Center's fortieth anniversary celebration in 1995.

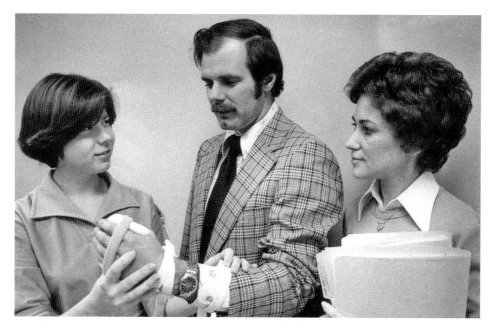

Dr. Thomas Freeland, center, was the first dean of the School of Health Related Professions. In 1977, the school entered into an agreement with Louisiana State University to train its students who wanted to study medical records in return for allowing Mississippi students to study occupational therapy. The reciprocal agreement was in place for several years. Now the school has its own OT program.

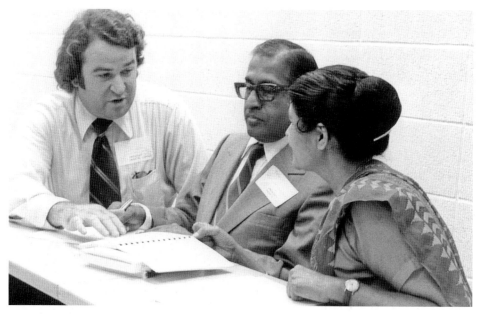

Jack Gordy, left, assistant dean of the School of Health Related Professions, also served a year as interim dean after the resignation of Dr. Maurice Mahan and before the appointment of Dr. Ben Mitchell. He's here at a meeting with pre-health professional advisors from the state's junior and senior colleges in the 1970s to help inform perspective students of the school's programs and requirements.

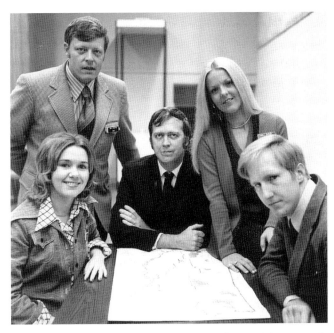

The first representatives of Project SNAP (Statewide Network of Allied Health Professions) included, from left, Cheryl Marble, Buck Whiffen, Dr. Ed King, Linda Butler, and Dr. David Allison. School of Health Related Professions dean Dr. Thomas Freeland devised the plan and applied for a successful grant to the VA Administration to fund it, one of the largest grants the Medical Center had received up to that time. The representatives covered the state visiting high schools and colleges to tell students about career opportunities in allied health.

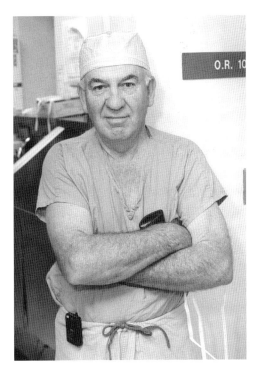

Dr. Norman C. Nelson made one of his most important appointments in 1976 in the person of Dr. Winfred L. Wiser as chair of obstetrics and gynecology. Wiser's twenty-year tenure turned around a languishing department and made it one of the most successful clinical departments at the Medical Center and one of the most sought-after ob-gyn residency programs in the country.

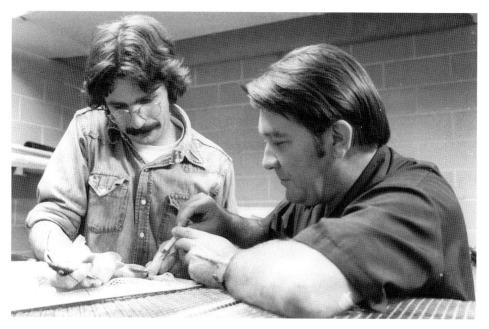

Dr. William Clem, right, chair of microbiology, was a key appointment in the graduate school. He came from Florida where he had studied the immune system in sharks and other salt-water fish. In Mississippi, he used farm-raised catfish as his experimental animals. His research was well funded, and Clem and his team made many important contributions to the field of immunology.

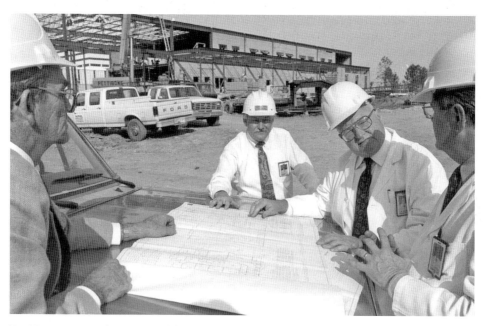

Dr. Norman C. Nelson, second from right, inspects plans for the new laundry building, a building project request Nelson took to the legislature for many years.

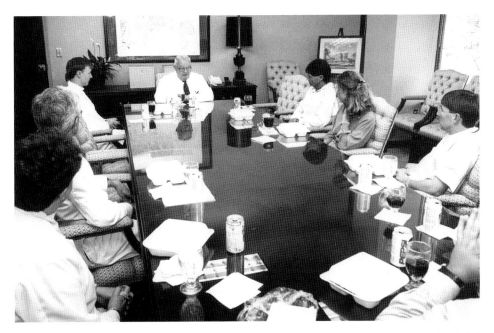

Dr. Norman C. Nelson liked to stay in close contact with students with regularly scheduled luncheons in his conference room.

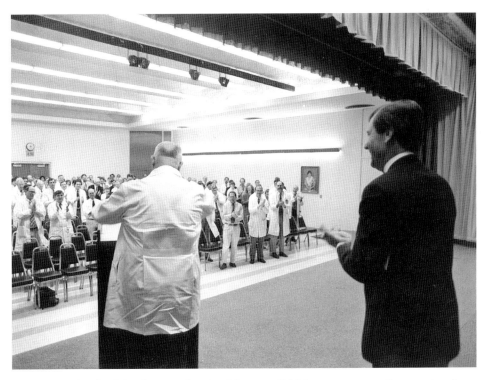

Presiding at his final faculty meeting, Dr. Norman C. Nelson gets a standing ovation from his faculty and from Chancellor Gerald Turner.

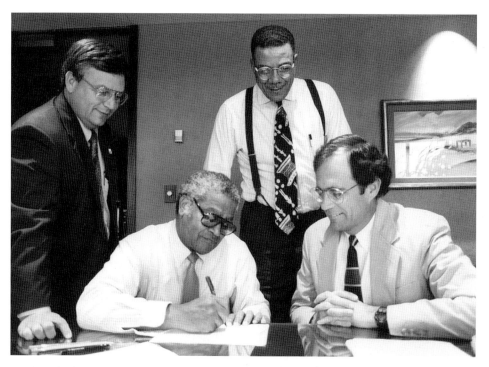

Signing the historic document that established the Jackson Medical Mall and the Jackson Medical Mall Foundation in 1995 are, from left, Ted Woodrell, University Hospital director, Dr. Aaron Shirley, Judge Rueben Anderson, and attorney Delbert Hoseman.

Dr. Patrick Sewell made international headlines with the first successful use of the interventional MRI to freeze and destroy kidney tumors in 1999. The procedure was first used on patients who faced the threat of having to have their one remaining kidney removed when their cancer recurred.

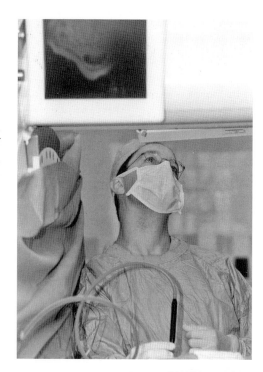

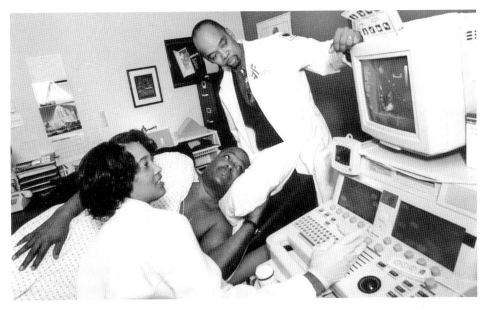

Jackson mayor Harvey Johnson Jr. volunteered to undergo the series of medical exams that participants in the Jackson Heart Study receive when they volunteer for the study. He did so to encourage African American residents to follow through with their own exams and to show they had nothing to fear. Dr. Herman Taylor is Jackson Heart Study director. Melanie Bradley is a cardiac sonographer. The Jackson Heart Study is the largest study ever undertaken to determine cardiovascular risk factors in African Americans.

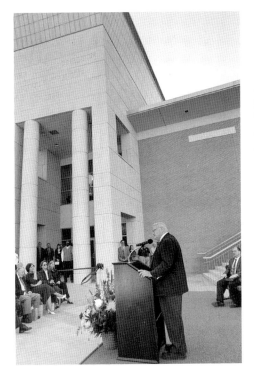

After a forty-four-year wait, the campus finally had a building just for students. The building dedication and formal opening in 1999 honored Dr. Norman C. Nelson, for whom the building is named.

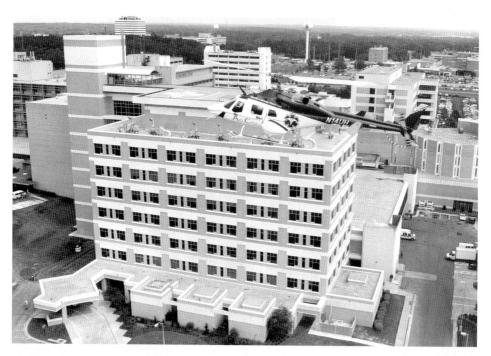

AirCare, the Medical Center's air ambulance, prepares to land on its helipad atop the Wallace Conerly Critical Care Hospital, which opened in 2001.

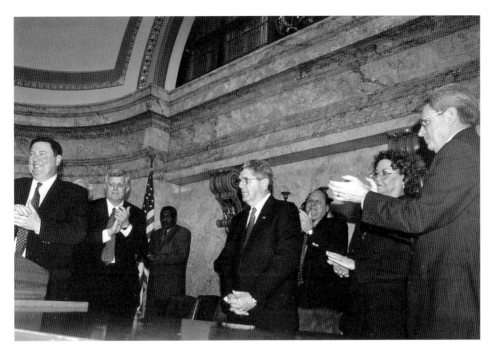

Dr. Wallace Conerly, center, was honored at Wally Conerly Day during a special session of the House of Representatives in 2003.

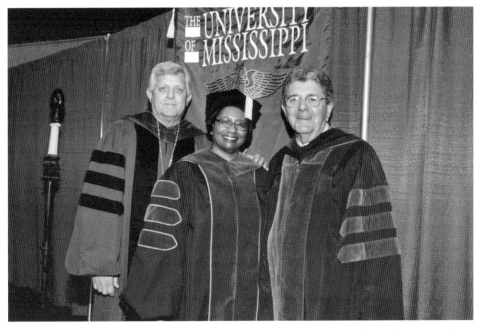

University chancellor Robert Khayat, left, and Medical Center vice chancellor Dr. Wallace Conerly greeted Dr. Ponjola Coney, commencement speaker in 2003. Coney is a graduate of the Medical Center and is now dean of the School of Medicine at Meharry Medical College in Nashville.

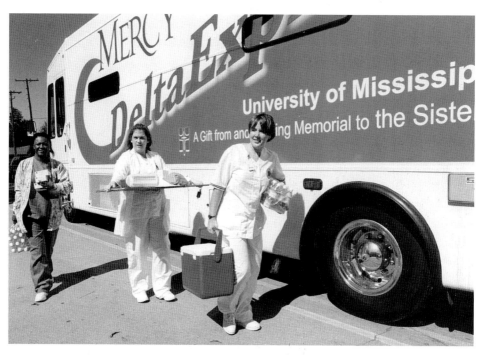

In 2003, the Sisters of Mercy of the Americas in Vicksburg donated their mobile health clinic and $50,000 to the School of Nursing. Dr. Peggy Hewlett, professor of nursing, spearheaded the project to provide health care to the state's rural poor. The Mercy Delta Express is fully equipped for medical and dental exams. Here, Dr. LaDona Northington, associate professor of nursing, and senior nursing students Jana Jordan and Jena Kilgo unload equipment for a stop at Mayersville.

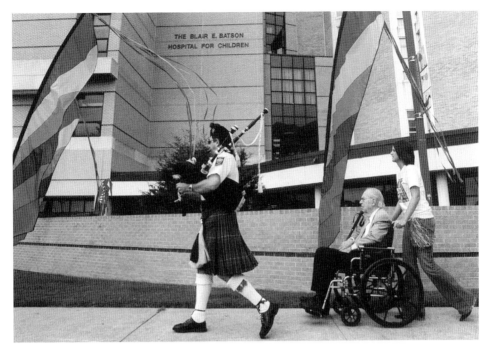

Piper Kris Carmichael leads the procession for the opening of the pediatric surgical center in 2004. For Dr. Blair E. Batson, in the wheelchair following the piper, this was the fourth major pediatric building project he has witnessed—the original children's hospital in 1968, the Mississippi Children's Cancer Clinic, the Blair E. Batson Hospital for Children in 1997, and the surgical center, which will provide complete surgical care from start to finish. Batson was the first chair of pediatrics.

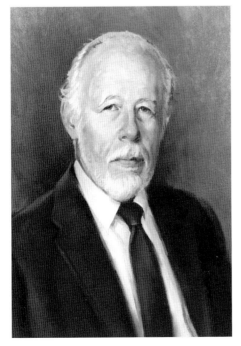

Dr. Sam Johnson headed ophthalmology at the Medical Center from 1955 until his death in 2000. The division became a department in 1987, and Johnson was named chair.

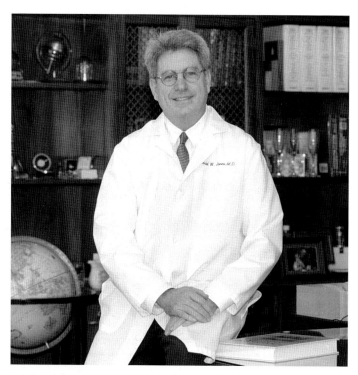

Dr. Daniel W. Jones is the Medical Center's seventh leader in its fifty-year history. With a major building program just completed, Jones wants to find new ways the Medical Center can help end disparities in health care.

Surgery nearly all of his career at the Medical Center. Ophthalmology and urology were the only exception. By 1960, anesthesiology and neurosurgery had already been made departments and beyond his control, much to Hardy's chagrin. The walk-out of the orthopedic residents in 1976 signaled the beginning of the end of orthopedics as a division within surgery. It became a department in 1986. Otolaryngology or ENT (ear, nose, and throat) surgery and plastic surgery had no problems with each other until the late 1970s. Hardy maintained that the fight between the two divisions didn't materialize at the Medical Center until both had full-time division directors (Dr. Godfrey Arnold in ENT and Dr. Michael Jabaley in plastic surgery) with fully accredited residency programs. Then the turf battles that were being played out all over the country began at the Medical Center.

Hardy wrote that he viewed his responsibility in the ENT-Plastic wars as preserving "a corpus of patient material for each specialty that would be essential to maintaining residency approval in all three disciplines." Hardy was clearly on the side of the plastic surgeons because of what he viewed as the continuing recalcitrance of the ENT residents and staff in disregarding the formal agreements between the two disciplines. "The ENT staff and residents were never satisfied," he wrote. "Each of the periodic meetings to agree upon allocations of turf resulted in a loss for plastic surgery." The final push came when the ENT residents performed face lifts (the "quintessence of Plastic Surgery," according to Hardy) at the neighboring VA Hospital.

Hardy wrote to Dr. Myron Lockey, the deputy director of the ENT division who intended to become the director at Arnold's retirement, that he may not be willing "to take on the Division . . . subject to the limitations which are going to be necessary to protect the legitimate interests of plastic surgery." He had written Arnold that residents whose names were listed on the schedule of procedures deemed to be the province of plastic surgery would be subject to cessation of pay, nonrenewal of contract, and problems with ultimate certification. The ENT residents threatened a lawsuit against Hardy (it never materialized or was dropped) for depriving them of surgical experiences necessary for learning their discipline.

By the time this conflict was being played out, Hardy was at the peak of influence in his profession. He was the ascending president of the most important surgical organization in the world, the American College of Surgeons. He was accustomed to the slings and arrows that came his way when he stood his ground. He had weathered the media storm and the professional criticism that followed the heart transplant in 1964 and had emerged as one of surgery's world leaders. Squabbling between divisions, and the animosity it generated among practitioners in town who took up for the ENT residents, was troubling, but not lethal.

Many viewed Hardy as authoritarian and monarchial. Dr. Mart McMullan readily admits there are a handful of the surgeons Hardy has trained who "despise him." McMullan, in his role as one of the founders of the Hardy Society (with fellow Hardy trainee Dr. Richard Yelverton), calls on surgeons who have been Hardy residents, and "two or three have told us they never want to see him again." Out of 140 total, McMullan doesn't see that as a bad percentage.

As much as McMullan admired and respected his mentor, he says Hardy was sometimes hard on his residents. "He was demanding, but I think it's fair to say that he never asked any resident to do anything he hadn't done in his own training or wasn't continuing to do during the course of being 'the professor.' He was always in the operating room or in the emergency room within minutes if we needed him, even if it was 2 A.M. He left such a lasting impression on me that I still think of him every day that I see and treat patients."

McMullan also recalls how Hardy made snap decisions—a necessity in the OR, but not always in administration. Sometimes those snap decisions were not in the department's best interests. He recalls one example in the brief tenure of the late Dr. Jeff Hollingsworth. "I know this story because after Jeff left the Medical Center, he was a partner in our practice. Jeff came from Stanford with outstanding credentials. Dr. Hardy had been very pleased to recruit him, and the department needed him. Dr. Hardy had promised Jeff that he would do everything he could to get a cardiac intensive care unit. Jeff had been there about a year, and there was still no ICU. Apparently, there had been some funding problems causing its delay. Jeff went to Dr. Hardy and told him he had seen nothing to indicate an ICU was even on the drawing board and that if he didn't see some progress within three months, he was leaving. Well, Dr. Hardy pushed his chair back, stood up, stuck out his arm to shake Jeff's hand, and said, 'Jeff, we certainly have enjoyed your time with us, and we wish you the very best.' With that, Jeff was gone, and the university lost a fine cardiac surgeon, but Dr. Hardy would not give in to threats."

McMullan, Yelverton, and the vast majority of Hardy's residents nearly all tell stories about how confident they were when they finished their training. In some cases, it surprised them that they were better prepared than their colleagues. "When I got to Mayo, I had already done a lot of surgery. Their residents only did a little assisting and gopher work in the first two years. We had a major role in surgery cases even in the first year. I was given responsibility at Mayo a little more quickly than others."

✳ ✳ ✳

After Hardy had retired from the Medical Center, he was often asked what he considered to be his greatest accomplishment. He never said it was in research, even in light of his historic operations. He did not count serving as an international leader in surgery as a major achievement. He considered his major achievement to be the training of surgeons for Mississippi. When he began to train students and residents in 1955, he said the entire state may have had two board certified surgeons in any field. Now any town of any size has several surgeons who are board certified, most of whom were trained by Hardy.

Many of his former students talk about how Hardy taught them to think and speak on their feet. It was common on rounds for Hardy to pepper the students and residents with questions, leaving the harder questions for the older residents. If someone faltered, Hardy told them to get their thoughts together, and he'd get back to them. "He was always polite, but demanding," recalled Dr. Richard Yelverton, also a Jackson surgeon, former student and resident of Hardy's, and founding member of the Hardy Society. McMullan said his fellow residents at Mayo were far more intimidated by questions from their mentor than he was. "It didn't bother me to be wrong. I had gotten used to it."

Dr. Johnnie Williamson of Tupelo spent a decade at the Medical Center as a student, a resident, and a fellow in vascular surgery, finishing in 1980. From Williamson's perspective, one of Hardy's notable achievements was that "he afforded good ole country boys from Mississippi the opportunity to become well-educated, well-trained professionals who could stand on our own wherever we wanted to go. On rounds, we went at breakneck speed, from the first floor to the top always using the stairs. We learned from his rapid-fire questioning how to think and talk on our feet. I learned later that ability was the mark of a Hardy-trained resident."

Dr. Ponjola Coney, one of fifteen African Americans to enroll in medical school at the Medical Center in 1974, also remembers Hardy as a staunch believer in oral questioning. "When I did my surgery block, he would make me stand right beside him in the OR. He told me that all his OR techs were black, and when we all got in the OR masked and gowned, he couldn't tell me from the techs. He said, 'I need to know where my students are.' It didn't offend me; he was just being honest. But the end result was, that because I was standing right by him, he constantly peppered me with questions throughout the entire operation. I was reading late into the night trying to read up on the complications and post-op care of any surgical case we might be in so I could be prepared. I was exhausted by the time the block was over." Coney graduated in 1978, then went to the University of North Carolina at Chapel

Hill for an ob-gyn residency. She is now the dean of the Meharry Medical College in Nashville. In the late 1970s, Hardy was still running up and down the stairs for rounds as he was in Yelverton's student days in the early 1960s. "He never, ever took the elevator. We ran up and down the stairs to get to patient rooms during rounds, and he never seemed breathless."

Hardy's youngest daughter, Dr. Katherine Hardy Little, offers a different perspective on the stair climbing. She says her father would fire off a question as soon as the group got to the top of the stairs and catch his breath while the student was answering the question. Katherine (known to friends and family as Kaky) is a gastroenterologist (digestive disease specialist) in Dallas, Texas. She was the only Hardy daughter to go to medical school in Jackson, although another sister, Julia, earned the MD at Harvard and practices psychiatry in Ann Arbor, Michigan. The oldest daughter, Louise Scott Roeska-Hardy, holds the PhD and teaches philosophy in Germany. Bettie W. Hardy also holds the PhD and is a clinical psychologist at the University of Texas, Southwestern.

In spite of all the obstacles to family life that his drive and ambition created, Hardy held to his family tightly, and he credited his wife, Weezie, for the love and stability she provided him and his daughters. And he made sure that in the time he had available, it was given to his family. Once in Jackson, his habit was to set his alarm for 3 A.M. He would have coffee and think about the surgical cases on schedule for the day. Then, until Weezie got up, he wrote either in longhand or by dictation, on a book or article. He would have a quick breakfast and be at the hospital by 7 A.M. for rounds or the first case.

Katherine Hardy remembers the coffee pot as "the major communication center of our home." Their father went to bed early, often before the girls had finished their homework for the next day. "Mom would leave him a note there asking that he wake her up at a certain time, or if we had a paper we wanted him to read before we had to turn it in, we'd leave it by the coffee pot. He would read it and leave us comments when he had his coffee, hours before we were up." While she was still in grade school (fourth or fifth grade), she had to write a report on apes. She dutifully went to the library and found a source book, wrote the paper, and left it at the coffee pot. The book that she relied on for information was Desmond Morris's *Naked Ape*, written not about apes, but about humans. It was one of the first works to treat humans as animals and to describe human behavior as a zoologist—which Morris was—would describe animal behavior. Morris goes into great detail about mating, courtship, and reproduction in humans, which the young author duly noted, thinking all the time, she said, "if apes do this, I wonder what humans do.

My father was shocked when he read the paper and asked me where I had gotten my information. When I told him, he just said perhaps I should leave out the details of the reproductive cycle."

Kaky, the youngest of the Hardy children, had been born in 1955 just before the Hardys moved to Jackson. Bettie was born in 1953. Julia was born in 1951, and the oldest daughter Louise was born in 1950.

Hardy did not make his job as chairman easier by being compliant. He moved quickly to establish his and the Medical Center's reputation, and he was impatient with those who didn't want to match his pace. McMullan said that Hardy once told him, "If you have a choice between having someone like you and respect you, take respect every time." Probably for that reason, Hardy says he had "few close friends." His family was an oasis, and the time he spent with his daughters and the love and respect he showed their mother left indelible impressions.

Katherine said her father took her to a farm to ride horses nearly every Saturday. "While I rode, he worked on a paper or read." Long after the girls left home, each kept a tiny garden wherever they were, perhaps to rekindle their childhood memories of the garden they grew with their father. Their father also loved music. He was always part of a band as a young man and in college, and he learned to play the piano. With the proceeds of his first book, he and Weezie bought a used piano to make the music to which his daughters and later his grandchildren would sing and dance. "On Sundays, we woke up to opera," Katherine said, "and once he took us all to the opera in New Orleans." When the girls were small, a Saturday ritual was spending their allowance at a local variety store. "We all got to travel with him, too. In the summer, he would take us with him wherever he was going to a meeting, and we got to see some incredible things."

When Weezie was diagnosed with a dementia (probably Alzheimer's) near the end of his career at the Medical Center, he turned his life over to her care. It was Weezie who, for the duration of their life together, had supported every move he made, encouraged him to follow his dreams as far as they would take him and remained steadfastly by his side through all the whirlwinds of his public life. Now, he would do the same for her. He would be by her side throughout the frightful loss of her self-hood. The daughters told McMullan the story of the Valentine dance at the Alzheimer's center where Weezie last lived. By this time Hardy himself was frail, but he had promised Weezie they would have a "date" every afternoon at 4 P.M. on what the staff at the center came to call the "Hardy love seat." Katherine said they would sit in front of the large picture window and talk, watch for deer, or just hold hands. One afternoon was the occasion of the Valentine's dance for the residents. The party had all but dispersed by 7 P.M., but the music was still playing, and Weezie was dancing with her "Jim." They danced and clung to each other long after the other guests had gone and the other residents put to bed. They danced as though their lives depended on each other, which in truth, they did.

Weezie died in 2000. Her "Jim" followed her in 2003.

Hardy's contributions to the Medical Center cannot be overstated, and it was the Medical Center's extreme good fortune for him to have chosen to spend his career in Mississippi. Few individuals could have accomplished what he did in the world arena; fewer still would have remained so focused on the daily pursuit of excellence in patient care and in teaching. And Hardy may have been right about his most important, although probably not his most impressive achievement: that of training hundreds of surgeons, like McMullan and Yelverton and Williamson, who think of him every day and still hold themselves accountable to his high standards.

CHAPTER 7

The Nelson Years: Building Excellence

By 1973, the Medical Center had achieved some remarkable feats. Dr. James Hardy, chairman of surgery, had pioneered organ transplantation. Dr. Arthur Guyton, chairman of physiology and biophysics, was spearheading research that was liberally funded by federal sources. Research on the artificial heart had culminated in a calf that lived twenty-six days with the silicone rubber model. A nurse-midwifery program was hailed nationally as a model to reduce infant mortality in rural areas, and Dr. John Bower had established one of the first artificial kidney units in the South. Two new schools were in the formative stages—Health Related Professions and Dentistry—and various faculty members throughout the Medical Center had distinguished themselves in national and international circles.

But progress came in very small increments. One of the worst recessions in the nation's history was wreaking havoc with many budgets, including the Medical Center's. Recruitment of faculty from outside the state was difficult because of the lingering negative perception of Mississippi brought on by the racial strife of the 1960s. The physical plant was quickly becoming outdated and overcrowded. The center was struggling with its limitations, and it would take a person of very special talents to wake the sleeping giant.

Who knew that the cheerful man with a crew cut from Louisiana State University would be that person? That bit of foresight can be attributed to Porter L. Fortune, University of Mississippi chancellor since 1968, and to Dr. Verner Holmes, the physician from McComb appointed by Governor J. P. Coleman to the Board of Trustees, Institutions of Higher Learning, in 1956. Fortune enlisted Holmes's help in identifying the individual who could shake the Medical Center from its lethargy. After a nationwide search, Fortune recommended Dr. Norman C. Nelson to the IHL board, which approved his appointment as vice chancellor for health affairs and dean of the School of Medicine.

The Medical Center's first leader, dean and director Dr. David Pankratz, had the gargantuan task of establishing the institution, laying the framework, putting systems in place. Dr. Robert Q. Marston, after Pankratz, spent much of his administrative energies in making sure the Medical Center was in compliance with new civil rights laws and regulations. Dr. Robert Carter, a pediatrician, stayed only three years, from 1967 until 1970. The hallmark of his administration was the initiation of the Mississippi Regional Medical Program. Dr. Robert E. Blount was dean and director until he retired in 1973, leaving the post that would be filled by Nelson. Blount had come to the Medical Center in 1968 as an assistant medical school dean after he retired from a thirty-five-year career in the army. Neither Carter nor Blount was at the helm long enough to turn the tide for the institution.

Pankratz, Marston, Carter, and Blount all initially held the titles of dean of the medical school and director of the Medical Center. Marston was named vice chancellor later in his tenure, and Nelson was the first person appointed as vice chancellor, a move that probably signaled a desire on Fortune's part to show Nelson's administrative link to the university campus. Nelson was the Medical Center's chief executive officer from 1973 until 1994. He brought to the post a rare combination of pragmatism and vision, and it wasn't long into his tenure before others at the Medical Center and in the community came to share his vision and appreciate his pragmatism. When Nelson retired in 1994, he refused offers to stay around and help run the place. He said he wanted to give his successor, Dr. Wallace Conerly, the freedom to make decisions without feeling as though his old boss was looking over his shoulder. At sixty-five, he said, "I've seen people stay in jobs long past their effectiveness, and I don't want to do that."

When Nelson arrived in July of 1973, he came to an institution that amounted to "city states" administratively. Without strong leadership at the top, some very strong-willed department chairs, most of whom had been in their jobs since 1955, ran their departments pretty much independently of the director's counsel. It would fall to Nelson to change that situation. And he wanted to change the orientation of those who still thought of the Medical Center as "the Ole Miss medical school." With four schools and a hospital, it was now a true academic health sciences center. It was the University of Mississippi Medical Center. He was also walking into several crises that had their origins in previous administrations. But for this and other challenges, he had prepared well.

Nelson was born in Hibbing, Minnesota, also the birthplace of singer and songwriter Bob Dylan. The Nelson family moved south, first to Vicksburg, Mississippi, where his father bought the National Park Hotel, and later to Texas. From Texas, he went to Louisiana and completed undergraduate and medical school at Tulane University in New Orleans, where he met and married Annie Lee Pitre, a Louisiana native.

He completed an internship and surgery residency at Charity Hospital in New Orleans, teaching hospital for Louisiana State University. During his residency, he became interested in surgical endocrinology and spent a year at Massachusetts General Hospital in Boston with Dr. Oliver Cope, a well-known endocrinologist. Nelson continued to do thyroid and parathyroid surgery up until he retired from the Medical Center in 1994. Back in New Orleans, he joined LSU's faculty and quickly became "an extremely valuable part of our teaching staff," according to Dr. Isidore Cohn, then chairman of the Department of Surgery at LSU. Cohn praised Nelson's work in setting up the surgical endocrinology service at LSU and Charity. "Norm's expertise in student teaching, resident instruction and pursuit of a clinical or experimental research problem made it clear that he was an outstanding individual," Cohn wrote in 1977 in support of Nelson's nomination for membership in the prestigious American Surgical Association.

Even as a young resident, Nelson was developing skills that would help him direct the Medical Center in Mississippi—skills recognized by Chancellor Fortune and Verner Holmes. In his ten years at LSU, he went from instructor in surgery, the lowest academic rank, to dean of the medical school. "When the time came to search for a new dean [for the LSU School of Medicine], he [Nelson] was the obvious choice and had the unusual distinction of being recommended by people in almost every department with whom he had ever had contact," Cohn said.

Early in his career, he almost gave up on academic medicine in favor of private practice. There's no doubt, he would have had a lucrative career. But Cohn talked him out of it. "I thought it would be a loss to academic surgery, and there's no question that I was right on that score. It was quite clear that he would be a superb surgery teacher and productive surgical researcher."

He was a Markle Scholar in Medicine from 1965 to 1970 under a program the foundation established in 1947 "in response to a need for more teachers, researchers and administrators in the nation's medical schools." The program awarded grants to "gifted" practitioners planning to further their career in academic medicine.

Having made the decision to stay in academic medicine, he maintained a dizzying pace of teaching and scholarship. He was named most inspirational teacher at LSU in 1966 and 1968, best clinical teacher in 1967, 1968, 1969, 1970, and 1971, and outstanding teacher of the senior class in 1970. He averaged publishing two papers a year for the ten years he was on the LSU faculty. One of those papers, "Portal and Peripheral Vein Immunoreactive Insulin before and after Glucose Infusion," published in the journal *Diabetes* in 1970, is considered "seminal" by some scientists. The paper, which Nelson coauthored with W. G. Blackard, "is the first I've seen that measured insulin and glucose concentrations in the portal vein," said Dr. Tom Coleman, a Medical Center professor emeritus of physiology whose company designs computer models of body function. Coleman explains that blood samples from the portal vein, the vessel that drains blood into the liver, can indicate what is coming out of the pancreas and the gastrointestinal tract and going into the liver. The problem is that the portal vein is difficult to access, but Nelson and his coauthor had done it successfully and delivered, in Coleman's terms, "excellent data." Coleman found Nelson's paper in 2004 when he was looking for a way to describe varying glucose concentrations in a computer simulation. "When I added the data from Nelson's paper, it worked perfectly."

But Nelson necessarily scaled back some of his teaching, surgery, and research activities when he came to Mississippi. Although he continued to do surgery and continued teaching in the form of lectures to students on thyroid and parathyroid disease, most of the scholarship he produced in Mississippi was the chapter on parathyroids in *Hardy's Textbook of Surgery*, edited by Dr. James D. Hardy, chairman of surgery. Running a medical center would require most of his energy and all of his talents.

One month after Nelson arrived in July of 1973, the chairperson of the Department of Psychiatry and Human Behavior resigned because of a very public debate about his credentials and the way he practiced psychiatry. Dr. Stewart Agras had been chairman of psychiatry since 1969. He came to Mississippi from the faculty of the University of Vermont where he had been highly regarded and well respected. An Englishman by birth, he was a Canadian citizen. He was licensed in Vermont and practiced in Mississippi in a reciprocal agreement, which was common. Agras had the full support of the Medical Center administration and members of the faculty, all of whom came to his defense when the General Legislative Investigating Committee (a "watchdog" group charged with investigating state agencies) targeted Agras at the request of a group of local mental health professionals.

The issue at the heart of the matter, according to state senator Theodore Smith of Corinth, was the failure of a local hospital to comply with its agreement with the Medical Center to allow medical students to rotate through its mental health center. Smith had written the minority opinion in the committee's report. Also at issue in the affair was the deep division in the profession of psychiatry between the Freudians and a growing faction of behaviorists, to which Agras belonged. While the Medical Center stood solidly behind Agras, it was not enough to keep Agras. He likely knew that such hostility from the local mental health community would derail many of his professional aspirations.

In 1973, Nelson was also walking into the very center of the storm in the national debate over a brain surgery procedure the mainstream press called "psychosurgery."

Dr. Orlando Andy, then chairman of the Department of Neurosurgery, had operated on a number of patients with great success in controlling extremely aggressive behavior or violent seizures. Unfortunately, Andy often saw his responsibility as limited to the patient and to science. He was not careful with paperwork, and documentation was not his strong suit. He became an easy target for groups who saw the procedure as a new form of lobotomy. The Mental Health Law Project was one such group. Officials from the group wrote to Robert Blount, Nelson's predecessor, in January of 1973 requesting that Blount provide them with existing policies and procedures governing Andy's work. Blount responded that Andy's work "has led to truly remarkable improvement in some 30 otherwise apparently hopeless cases exhibiting medically uncontrollable self-destructive or criminally aggressive behavior." He explained that a peer review committee had existed for some time, but new protocols were being discussed and a new committee was being formed for development of such protocols.

In early July of 1973, just days before Nelson would arrive in the vice chancellor's post, an attorney representing the Mental Health Law Project succeeded in getting an injunction that would prevent Andy from performing surgery already scheduled at the Medical Center. The patient was a child, and the parents wanted her to have the surgery, fearing that she would harm herself or others during violent seizures. Andy agreed not to do the surgery rather than force a showdown.

The storm abated somewhat after Nelson arrived on campus. Apparently, Andy was persuaded of the necessity of better documentation, and the new committee had to approve all his protocols. In 1978, he began implanting electrodes in the brain instead of making a surgical incision. That innovation greatly reduced the controversy because nothing irreversible was done to the brain. The patient stimulated the electrodes whenever he or she needed relief from a particular symptom. Later on, Andy's duties as department chair would be taken away from him. Andy had a brilliant mind that was fascinated with the relationship of brain function to behavior. He was far ahead of the rest of the scientific community in exploring the potential of the brain, and much of his early work has been validated by scientists and neurosurgeons working today, but his intense interest in research often overshadowed his interest in running a department.

Andy was one of the original faculty members who were still around when Nelson arrived on July 15, 1973. Others were department chairs Blair Batson (pediatrics), Warren Bell (clinical laboratory sciences), Arthur Guyton (physiology), James Hardy (surgery), Tom Brooks (preventive medicine), Louis Sulya (biochemistry),

Robert Sloan (radiology), Thomas Blake and Herbert Langford (medicine), Don Turner (surgery), Lucy Lawson (microbiology), Jack Crowell (physiology), and Forest Hutchison (preventive medicine). Other old-timers included Charles Randall, second chairman of microbiology, appointed in 1957; Lane Williams, second chairman of anatomy, appointed in 1958; Harper Hellems, chairman of medicine, appointed in 1965 after the death of the first medicine chair, Robert Snavely; Joel Brunson, chairman of pathology since 1959; Richard Klein, acting chairman of pharmacology, appointed to the faculty in 1959. James Arens had been chairman of anesthesiology since 1972. Henry Thiede, chairman of ob-gyn, succeeded the first ob-gyn chair Michael Newton in 1967. Wilfred Gillis, chairman of the new Department of Family Medicine, was appointed in 1973. James Suess had been a member of the faculty since 1962, and Nelson chose him as acting chair of psychiatry in the wake of Agras's resignation. Dr. Thomas E. Freeland had come the year before Nelson arrived to become dean of the newly formed School of Health Related Professions. Dr. Wallace V. Mann, the new dean of the School of Dentistry, which would enroll its first students in 1975, began his duties on January 1, 1974.

One of the first administrative changes Nelson made was the appointment of two associate deans. They were Dr. Carl Evers, associate medical school dean for student affairs, and Dr. Henry Thiede, associate dean for academic affairs. It fell to Thiede to assign order to the chaos of postgraduate training at the Medical Center. In medical schools and teaching hospitals, the residents are neither fish nor fowl, but they're both students and employees. The clinical department chairs had established residency training in their own fields as their needs arose, and there was really no central office that kept track of all the residents. Collectively, the interns, residents, and fellows (all those in further training beyond the MD) in a teaching hospital are the "housestaff." In September of 1973, Thiede wrote Nelson that "reliable data on housestaff is impossible to find. One person in medical school administration needs to be totally responsible for coordinating, supervising and approving all house staff appointments, salaries, changes in program, funding, affiliations, etc." Thiede was that person until he resigned a year later. Nelson named Dr. Richard Miller, a highly respected pediatric surgeon, as associate dean and gave him the responsibility of organizing and keeping track of the Medical Center's housestaff programs. Evers served as associate dean until his death in 1992 from injuries sustained in a bicycle accident.

Another change Nelson made was to create divisions of Continuing Health Professional Education and Learning Resources. Continuing education for health professionals was becoming vastly more important than it was when the Medical

Center began in 1955. It needed a full-time director and staff of its own. Nelson tapped Dr. Roland B. Robertson, who would later become chief-of-staff at the VA Medical Center and still later associate vice chancellor under Wallace Conerly, as director of continuing education. The Division of Learning Resources would allow the Medical Center to apply for federal grant money that was available for improvement of health professional instruction through the use of new communication technologies.

Judging from media reports in the early months of Nelson's tenure, there were other issues that demanded his attention. The Medical Center was only eighteen years old, and its pace of supplying physicians for the state wasn't fast enough if editorials in state newspapers were any indication. An editorial in the *Tupelo Daily Journal* in February 1974 noted that the medical school had accepted only 117 students the previous year in the face of increased demand for physicians in Mississippi. The editorial called on the legislature to increase its commitment to the school. The Mississippi Economic Council urged the "rapid expansion in family medicine at the Medical Center" to further address the problem of getting physicians into rural areas, and officials from the Mississippi State Medical Association also pointed to a physician shortage.

Nelson was keenly aware of the health care needs of the state, its need for health professionals, and the Medical Center's crucial role in meeting that need. "It was always about students with him," said Brenda Melohn, now the associate vice chancellor for institutional affairs but the institution's chief financial officer for much of Nelson's tenure. She worked with Nelson from 1976 until he retired in 1994. "Behind every decision he made was his focus on what he considered to be the primary mission of the Medical Center, the education of health professionals. Would it enhance our educational mission? If we ever forgot that or got impatient with some student issue that may have sounded trivial to us, he was always the one to remind us that students were our reason to be."

In response to the state's need, he made the decision to increase the entering medical school class size to 150 for the 1974 fall class. The previous year, the school had admitted 122 in the freshman class, up from 117 the year before. Also in response to medical manpower needs, the Department of Family Medicine, after approval from the Residency Review Committee, increased the number of its first-year slots from four to sixteen beginning July 1, 1974.

The Medical Center's 1974–1975 appropriation from the state legislature jumped to $16 million up from $12 million the year before. It was Nelson's first budget pitch to the legislature, and he got a 33 percent increase from the year before. It was this budget increase that allowed the Medical Center to increase the entering medical school class to 150. And it was just a token of things to come in Nelson's twenty-one-year relationship with the body that would determine the Medical Center's future. Nelson applied all of his talents as a communicator to his dealings with the legislature. Dr. John Rupert Lovelace, a member of the IHL board when Nelson was appointed, says Nelson "captured the interest of state leaders with his enthusiasm and optimism about medicine in Mississippi. For twenty-one years, his audience remained captivated by his knowledge, his skill, and his deep commitment to the Medical Center and to the state."

Dr. Wallace Conerly, the person who succeeded Nelson as vice chancellor when Nelson retired in 1994, said Nelson "established a credibility with the legislature that lasted his whole tenure and extended to mine and to that of Dan Jones." Much of that credibility came from Nelson's steel-trap mind that never forgot a figure or obscure fact about the institution he oversaw. He could tell legislators how many employees were in the housekeeping department, how many square feet the laundry needed, or how much a hospital wing renovation would cost to heat and cool. Marjorie Solomon, who was the Medical Center's chief budget officer, went with Nelson to the legislature when he presented the budget. "He understood budget matters better than anyone I've ever worked with who wasn't a CPA. My job was to give him the information, then he presented it to the legislature in his own fashion. He never got a figure wrong, even if it was one you gave him last year. He always told them the truth, even if he thought it might hurt the Medical Center's chances to get the best appropriation. They appreciated it and came to trust what he said."

Nelson enjoyed the legislature, and the lawmakers, in turn, enjoyed him. Conerly said it was because there was never any show of arrogance in Nelson's demeanor. "He never represented himself as more sophisticated, better educated, or smarter than they, and he never hinted that the Medical Center was a superior institution, only that it had a unique mission in higher education in Mississippi." Nelson had a relationship with the legislature that was rare for a budget supplicant, and it paid off for the Medical Center. Solomon recalled a time when she went with Nelson to the legislature after he had lost a great deal of weight in an attempt to avoid hip replacement surgery. "Naturally they all asked him about it, about how much weight he had lost, and how he had done it. He had on a belt that he wore when he was about twice the size he was then and had it wrapped it around him twice. I'm sure he wore it that day knowing they would ask about it. But he opened his coat and showed them his belt and stretched it out. He told them he wasn't sure how many pounds he'd lost, but that he'd lost 'this much' in belt size. I never heard them laugh as loudly as they did then."

It wasn't all rosy with the legislature, even for a master communicator. In 1977, Senator Bill Burgin, who was chairman of the appropriations committee, accused Nelson of having a "slush fund" in the amount of $700,000 and thought the Medical Center's request for money for maintenance and upkeep on the new clinical sciences building was audacious. "The erroneous charge by Dr. Nelson that funds were not appropriated to operate this facility is clearly specious when this $700,000 slush fund is considered," Burgin fumed. The money was "overhead"—the money in grant funds that is set aside to pay for fiscal facilities, space, and utilities to conduct the project for which the grant is awarded. The federal government has a formula to calculate overhead. The IHL board hired a CPA firm to investigate the Medical Center's budget figures, and their opinion was that the Medical Center had used accepted methods of determining the overhead amount and that it could not be used for anything other than expenses incurred for a particular grant.

That sort of thing didn't happen many times in Nelson's years of appearing before the legislature, and Nelson won a decisive victory in 1986 in getting the legislature to approve a consolidated budget for the Medical Center. Until that time, each school, the hospital, and the Medical Center support services had a separate line-item budget with budget amounts strictly divided into categories. Any movement of funds from one category to another had to be approved by the IHL board. The year 1986 was a particularly tight budget year, and Nelson apparently persuaded Representative Ed Perry that the necessary cuts to the Medical Center budget wouldn't hurt nearly so much if the Medical Center had budgetary control over the money it got from the legislature. It was the first state agency to get such an appropriation, and in Conerly's estimation, it "saved our bacon."

In the decade of the 1980s, the Medical Center faced several budget crises that Nelson managed in his own way. Some programs suffered to the point of extinction, such as the highly regarded clinical pastoral education program to train clergy in the pastoral care of hospitalized patients, training that is required by nearly every seminary. In turn, the Medical Center patients had access to the chaplains, who were liked and appreciated by the patients and staff. Other programs were cut and later revived, such as the helicopter emergency transport service. Nelson also eliminated several hundred positions. It was his opinion that it was better to cut entire programs than to make cuts across the board. He wanted to maintain excellence in programs that related directly to teaching, according to Brenda Melohn, the chief financial officer. Budget restrictions in the 1980s partly accounted for the decrease in the medical school class size, which had been increased to 150 in 1974. The Liaison Committee on Medical Education (LCME) of the American Medical Association, the organization that the medical school looks to for accreditation, has to approve any enlargement of class size, which it did in 1974. In later site visits, LCME representatives said the school's physical and personnel resources couldn't accommodate 150 students per year. In the bad budget years of the 1980s, the entering class size was gradually decreased.

While steadily gaining credibility with the lawmakers, Nelson and other higher education leaders in the state faced the continuing problem of compliance with federal guidelines for desegregation. Just months into his new job, Nelson served on a committee with other IHL heads to prepare a plan for the IHL board to submit to the Department of Health, Education, and Welfare, the forerunner of the Department of Health and Human Services, for the further desegregation of the state's colleges and universities. Others on that committee from the Medical Center were Peter Stewart, the director of minority student affairs, and Dr. Helen Barnes, an African American ob-gyn who was on the Medical Center faculty. The plan, submitted by the board in February 1973, was unacceptable to the Black Mississippians' Council on Higher Education, who countered with its own plan, naming the Medical Center specifically. This group wanted Jackson State University to have administrative authority over the Medical Center, a foreshadowing of a suit to be filed that would last throughout Norman Nelson's entire tenure and beyond.

The Ayers case was filed by a group of black Mississippians in 1975, claiming that Alcorn, JSU, and Mississippi Valley State had been denied equal distribution of the state's financial resources and were historically underfunded compared to the state's historically white colleges. The suit went through many courts, including the United States Supreme Court. Finally, in 2004, the Fifth District Court of Appeals upheld the settlement of $503 million the legislature must appropriate for the historically black colleges and universities in Mississippi. In early 2004, with most of the original plaintiffs willing to accept the settlement, plaintiff attorney Alvin Chambliss Jr. was considering an appeal.

While the whole idea of the suit was to strengthen the historically black colleges and universities, the plaintiffs sought also to switch administrative authority for the Medical Center from the University of Mississippi to Jackson State University, a suggestion that never materialized.

As the Medical Center's vice chancellor, Nelson's role in these kinds of issues was a collaborative one with other institution heads. For other administrative challenges, Nelson sought support and advice from faculty and the chancellor. In July 1976, Nelson was confronted with a situation that threatened an entire program of patient care and training at the Medical Center. The conflict illustrates much about how Nelson made decisions as well as what he valued and what he didn't. Nelson preserved his own account of what happened during the walkout of the orthopedic residents that began on July 7, 1976.

Nelson was at a budget commission meeting when attorney William Winter, later to become governor, called him asking for a meeting with him. Nelson said he couldn't leave and asked Winter if he could come there. He did, accompanied by the chief resident in orthopedics, Pat Barrett, who was acting as a spokesperson for the group of residents who were unhappy with their chief, Dr. Paul Derian, chief of the Division of Orthopedics in the Department of Surgery. Barrett enumerated fourteen concerns about the leadership of Derian, whom the residents wanted Nelson to dismiss. The one that most concerned Nelson was the charge that Derian charged for patient care rendered by residents when he was not present. He told Barrett this was of "grave concern" to him, but that he had to have proof of wrongdoing before he could consider dismissal. He did offer to make a temporary change in the division leadership until all the facts were gathered. Apparently this was not what the residents wanted, and Barrett gave Nelson a letter of resignation that contained signatures of all the residents. Derian voluntarily stepped down as division chief and took three weeks of leave time. He was granted sabbatical leave from September 1, 1976, to March 1, 1977, then put on unpaid leave. In July 1977, Derian agreed to submit his resignation. He did not, and so his contract expired. He never came back to the Medical Center, and none of the residents returned. Dr. Frazier Ward accepted the position as interim chief of the division on September 1, 1976, and Dr. James L. Hughes became permanent chief of the division on January 1, 1977. The division became a department in 1986 with Hughes as chairman. Hughes and his faculty (including Ward, who stayed on the faculty) turned the department into one of the best-run, most successful departments at the Medical Center. Its residency program is still one of the most sought after in the country.

This is what can be learned about how Nelson made decisions. He weighed conflicting information from both sides—well-respected members of the faculty who said they had never seen Derian act inappropriately as well as respected orthopedic surgeons in town who supported the residents and thought they were showing courage in walking out. He didn't like ultimatums, nor did he appreciate the residents hiring an attorney before they talked to anyone at the Medical Center. "I tried to keep the lines of communications open between me and the housestaff," he told the executive faculty. "I meet every week with the president of the Housestaff Association." Nelson also balked at the residents trying to exert pressure by having their attorney call individual members of the IHL board, the president of the Medical

Alumni Chapter, and others in the community. At one point Winter called Dr. Verner Holmes, the IHL board member from McComb, to see if he would intercede on behalf of the residents. Holmes, once again showing how much faith he had in Nelson's administration, told Winter he would not meet with the residents and he wouldn't intercede because he knew Nelson would make the decision that would be best for the Medical Center. Holmes did call Nelson to let him know that Winter had called him, but stayed out of the fray. Finally, Nelson thought the residents had acted irresponsibly in walking out on their patients, showing no regard for either patients or the institution. He conceded that the residents were all good physicians who had acted as they had because of fear of reprisal from Derian, and he gave them credit for the work they completed while they were in the residency program. With Derian out of the picture, the residents insisted they all be taken back as a group, but Nelson would not consider it. Each of them would be considered individually.

Meanwhile, crisis intervention was just a tiny fraction of life at the Medical Center during the second half of the 1970s. The first four residents in the new Department of Family Medicine finished their training in 1976, all prepared to practice in Mississippi towns. Family medicine, established at the Medical Center in 1973, was part of a national resurgence of interest. In the late 1960s and early 1970s, the nation found itself with a plethora of specialists but few generalists. The old general practitioners who finished medical school before the age of specialization and whose postgraduate training consisted of a year of a rotating internship were dying or retiring, and there were no young doctors to fill the gap. Family medicine was an oxymoron, a "specialty" in general practice. It offered medical school graduates three years of training to be the front lines of medical practice. The department at the Medical Center aligned itself with family physicians throughout the state who volunteered to teach medical students in their offices so that the students could experience family medicine as it was practiced in small towns and rural areas. In turn, it gave the preceptors the option of becoming board certified in family medicine through a series of continuing education courses. The creation of the department was a response to the state's need for physicians who would practice away from the urban areas and take care of patients in all sections of the state. Dr. Wilfred Gillis was the first department chair to resign in 1986. His successor was an early resident of the family medicine program, Dr. Melessa D. Phillips, who is still chair of the department, the first woman to chair a department in the School of Medicine.

In 1975, Nelson made a key appointment in the person of Dr. Winfred L. Wiser. He became chairman of the Department of Obstetrics and Gynecology on May 1, 1976, just two months before the orthopedic walkout. Wiser inherited a languishing department with only five full-time faculty members and only half its residency slots filled. The departmental budget was $284,000 and there was no money for research. In just months, he had recruited a highly productive, committed faculty, which in turn made recruitment of residents easier. He also worked quickly to establish a research endowment, a move that enhanced recruitment because it showed that the department was committed to research even if federal dollars weren't immediately available. He stepped down as department chairman in 1996. By 1999, when the Winfred L. Wiser Hospital for Women and Infants was dedicated in his honor, the annual budget for the department was $3.8 million, with a research endowment for his department alone at $3 million.

Growing student enrollment was a happy problem for Nelson. Early in his tenure, Nelson had encouraged a young teacher in the nursing school to apply for the dean's post when Christine Oglevee retired. Dr. Edrie George reluctantly did so, and was chosen by the search committee and approved by Nelson. One of her first accomplishments was to compress the school's curriculum from three years to two, taking advantage of the state's excellent junior college system (or other four-year colleges) where nursing students completed the first two years of the baccalaureate curriculum. The school could then eliminate some of the duplication of courses and concentrate all the nursing coursework in the last two years. That one change greatly enhanced the enrollment in the School of Nursing. Enrollments were also increasing in the School of Health Related Professions (SHRP) as programs were added or enhanced. The first dental students began classes in 1975, further increasing student numbers. Medical school enrollment in the class entering in 1977 was 152. Resources were strained.

Dr. W. Lane Williams, chairman of the Department of Anatomy, was trying to make scarce cadavers go around. When Jack Gordy, assistant dean of the School of Health Related Professions, appealed to Williams for a cadaver for the physical therapy students, Williams responded: "At UMC during the past ten years, student use of cadavers has doubled while the supply has decreased. I see no indication for improvement of the situation." Nelson approved the transfer of one cadaver to SHRP even in the face of cadaver shortages. Dental, medical, and physical and occupational therapy students, as well as surgery residents, all use human cadavers as part of their medical training. For many years, there was a critical shortage, but changing ideas and attitudes among the public, as well as a well-developed body donation program, headed by Dr. Tony Moore in anatomy, have succeeded in making cadavers plentiful.

It was no surprise to anyone that Nelson was personally involved in a dispute over cadavers. He was involved in nearly everything. His dual role of vice chancellor, literally the CEO of the Medical Center, and dean of the School of Medicine, meant that administrative authority was very centralized. Nearly everyone has criticized the structure, even the editor of the *Northside Sun*, a Jackson weekly newspaper. Accrediting agencies say it puts too much authority in one person; people who study management say it's a bad idea to have so many people answering to one person. And yet, with Norman Nelson it worked. It worked because he could remember everything about what everyone was doing, and he hardly ever spent time away from the Medical Center. Melohn said he went to one dean's meeting of the Association of American Medical Colleges during his twenty-one-year tenure, but found it "a waste of time." He made time to attend any event at the request of state or local officials, the medical community, and community groups who wanted him to speak about the Medical Center, and any event he was invited to by Chancellor Fortune or Gerald Turner (the Ole Miss chancellor who succeeded Fortune). He just as assiduously avoided most other invitations, especially lavish drug-company-sponsored events or elaborate receptions for deans and their spouses. He hated travel, with the possible exception of weekend trips to New Orleans where the Nelsons indulged their hobby of collecting art and antiques. As a result, he was probably more physically present than any other dean in the country.

"The Medical Center was small enough in the early days of his administration that he could do that," said Conerly. "And although the titles are still there in the one person, vice chancellor and dean, I delegated much more than Norman did, and Dan [Dan Jones, Conerly's successor] delegates more than I did. The growing complexity of the institution requires it."

Both Chancellor Fortune and Chancellor Turner appreciated Nelson's ability to run the Medical Center yet keep them in the loop about what was going on 160 miles south of Oxford. "Norman and I had one of the most complementary administrative styles I ever hope to be associated with," said Turner, now president of Southern Methodist University. "When I was appointed chancellor in 1984, I told him I had no intention of trying to do his job. I did, however, tell him I wanted to discuss issues and decisions that had implications beyond the campus. He never deviated from that understanding, and it was a mutually satisfying relationship. As his day progressed, he kept a list of topics to discuss with me, and it was always ready when I would call. I enjoyed working with him tremendously."

Nelson and Fortune also enjoyed a very close relationship, characterized by deep friendship and mutual respect. Perhaps the only time Nelson failed to let Fortune know what was going on during a crisis was during the orthopedic residents' walkout. Fortune was having heart surgery at the time, and Nelson declined to give him information that would worry him.

Nelson's talents as a communicator were put to good use in dealing with strong-willed, persuasive department chairs who were accustomed to having things go their way. Nelson's successor, Wallace Conerly, who worked side by side with Nelson for twelve years, says Nelson just "talked them down." He recalled one meeting of the long-range planning committee, an institutional committee that decided the priorities for campus expansion, in which Nelson was trying to bring Dr. Arthur Guyton, chairman of physiology and biophysics, around to his way of thinking about a campus project. "He knew Guyton was opposed to it, and he just out-talked Dr. Guyton. We sat in that meeting for two or three hours with Dr. Nelson going on in his eloquent way, and he absolutely turned Dr. Guyton around. That was the only time I had ever seen anyone dissuade Dr. Guyton from a position he held. It was always the gospel according to Guyton. But Dr. Nelson did it." Dr. James Hardy, the chairman of surgery, was a bigger challenge for Nelson. "Both were surgeons; both had very strong egos; and they challenged each other, up to the very end of Dr. Hardy's tenure. Hardy had his own empire and didn't want anyone intruding on it," Conerly said. Nelson, however, knew the importance of Guyton and Hardy to the Medical Center and to the state. He recommended to the IHL board that both be honored with buildings named for them.

One of Nelson's greatest challenges in the 1970s was the need to improve the physical plant. Enrollment was steadily increasing, and patient care numbers were spiraling. In 1974, the original clinics, built in 1955, recorded 68,000 clinic visits in space designed for a maximum of 50,000 annually. Labor and delivery in the hospital was still in its 1955 space. As Winfred Wiser streamlined his department and improved the care of women and babies in the state, deliveries in the hospital, already outstripping the 1955 capacity, grew even more. In the early 1980s, conditions were so crowded in labor and delivery, that many women in labor had to wait in a hallway bed. The emergency room, still in its 1955 space, was straining at the seams with a growing number of trauma cases.

In the eighteen years before Nelson arrived on campus, additions to the original complex included the nursing education building (the Oglevee Building, named for the school's first dean, later to be significantly enlarged during Conerly's tenure), a dormitory each for men and women students, married student apartments, a research wing, the hospital's south wing, and a round children's hospital. During Nelson's tenure, the School of Dentistry, a walkway connecting it to the research wing, a major classroom addition, and the clinical sciences wing (later named the

James D. Hardy Clinical Sciences Building) opened in 1977. In 1983, the acute services wing opened, tripling the space for the emergency department, surgery, and intensive care. That same year, a new library and learning resources building opened. The pavilion, a free-standing clinic where physicians on faculty could see private patients, opened in 1987. The Ronald McDonald House, where the families of patients in the children's hospital can be housed during a child's illness, opened in 1989. The Mississippi Children's Cancer Clinic opened in 1991. It provided the foundation for the Blair E. Batson Hospital for Children, completed in 1997. The old laundry, virtually destroyed by the shifting of the Yazoo Clay beneath it, was replaced in 1992. In 1993, the Arthur C. Guyton Laboratory Research Building opened.

As the learning resources building (which would also house the Rowland Medical Library) was nearing completion, Nelson realized he had the opportunity to honor the man who had been so crucial in the Medical Center's development during his twenty-four-year tenure on the Board of Trustees, Institutions of Higher Learning. The IHL board granted Nelson's request to name the new building for Dr. Verner S. Holmes. He was appointed by Governor J. P. Coleman, a staunch supporter of the Medical Center, who was persuaded that a physician on the IHL board would better understand the needs of this medical center that was unique in Mississippi's scheme of higher education. Holmes, who had the distinction of serving longer than any other board member—two consecutive terms—gave invaluable aid and assistance to a succession of Medical Center administrators. It was the second building on campus named in honor of an individual. The original medical school building was named for Dean David Pankratz several years after Pankratz died.

The University Medical Pavilion replaced the North Clinic, a tiny space in the original medical school wing where faculty saw private patients. As the faculty grew, and as town physicians grew less resistant to the idea of medical school faculty having private patients, new space was demanded. It was essential that the teaching hospital attract patients who were covered by insurance. The more paying patients the hospital could attract, the more revenues the hospital provided to help defray the cost of running the Medical Center. A facility that was easy for patients to access, with front-door parking, was desperately needed. After Nelson named Conerly his assistant vice chancellor, he put him in charge of overseeing campus construction projects. When they began to talk about the need for a new private practice clinic, Chancellor Fortune almost simultaneously was renewing his acquaintance with Dr. Thomas Frist Sr., the founder of the giant Hospital Corporation of America (HCA, later Quorum Health Services). Frist, a native of Meridian, was a graduate of the two-year medical school in Oxford. He and Fortune were discussing ways he could help his alma mater, and Fortune introduced him to Nelson and Conerly. As a result, the University of Mississippi Medical Center and Hospital Corporation of America formed one of the most unusual alliances in medical education. As Conerly describes the progression of events, the partnership came about because of the needs of the Medical Center and the soft spot Frist had for Mississippi. "We were losing our hospital director, Bill Newell, to the Yale New Haven Hospital, and the pay for hospital directors had increased substantially across the country. We knew we probably could not afford a first-rate director with what we were able to pay. But more important, we were about to lose Medicare funds because we didn't have the computers necessary to fill out the new forms Medicare was about to come out with. At that time, all state agencies were under the Central Data Processing Authority, and we couldn't even buy a computer without their okay. We knew if we couldn't come up with something, it would be disastrous for us."

What the two parties came up with was the management services contract between the hospital and the HCA (now Quorum). For an annual fee paid by the hospital, Quorum supplies three or four key personnel in hospital administration, including the hospital director, and allows the hospital to purchase supplies under using the same bulk purchasing rate as all the hospitals Quorum owns, amounting to substantial savings. "What we save every year as a member of their purchasing group more than pays for our contract fee with them," Conerly said. In the then-immediate crisis of computer upgrades, HCA supplied the computers so the hospital could comply with Medicare demands. Quorum also agreed to build the pavilion as another shot in the arm to the hospital. Built at a cost of $5 million, the Medical Center bought it from Quorum for $1.2 million several years later and doubled its size. Skeptics often ask what Quorum gets out of the management services agreement, and the simple answer is, according to Conerly, that Frist honored his allegiance to his home state and the university with his gift, and Quorum gets to name a teaching hospital in its affiliation list. When the Medical Center announced the contract in 1984, HCA owned 172 hospitals and managed 174 others.

Both the Ronald McDonald House and the Mississippi Children's Cancer Clinic were paid for with private donations from the community. The Junior League of Jackson raised the funds for the cancer clinic. League volunteers provided extra help for pediatric cancer patients when the patients were seen with all the other pediatric clinic patients in the old children's hospital. Cancer patients are more prone to infections spread by contact with other children, and these infections in cancer patients that might be mildly annoying to healthy children can be severe or even life-threatening. League volunteers saw the need for a separate clinic and persuaded the organization to take on the task of raising the money for it.

Nelson lobbied the legislature for a new laundry almost from the beginning of his tenure. It took nearly twenty years, but it was finally a reality in 1992. Marjorie Solomon, his budget director, said he was "passionate" in his appeal to the legislature. "He would describe the deplorable conditions laundry workers had to endure, how it was being propped up literally, how it should be condemned." Solomon said when the legislature finally voted to approve funds for the construction, one of them rose to say, "The only reason we're appropriating funds for this laundry is that we're sick and tired of hearing you ask for it."

Another story, unconfirmed by former lieutenant governor Brad Dye, but told by Rupert Lovelace, a member of the IHL board, has Dye promising Nelson money for a laundry as Dye is being wheeled into the operating room after having a less-than-comforting preoperative chat about Dye's chances of recovery.

Even though the legislature did eventually come up with money for the laundry, it was apparent to Nelson that many other desperately needed construction projects would go unfunded waiting for state revenues. The Medical Center would have to come up with other ways of paying for most of its needs. The Department of Obstetrics and Gynecology had received additional hospital space by renovating areas that adjoined labor and delivery. By the late 1980s, the department's physicians, who were specialists in the treatment of pregnancies that could endanger the life of the mother or the baby (called high-risk pregnancies), were delivering nearly five thousand babies annually in space designed for twenty-five hundred. And more than 70 percent of those deliveries were high risk, requiring more staff, more equipment, and more space than normal deliveries. A perinatal center was a perennial on the Medical Center's most-needed construction list, but the likelihood of state appropriations for it dimmed with each budget cycle. Brenda Melohn, the center's chief financial officer, said the establishment of the nonprofit Medical Center Educational Building Corporation (MCEBC) in 1991 solved that dilemma and paved the way for making possible the largest building program in the history of higher education in Mississippi. Earlier, the state had passed legislation that would allow state agencies to borrow money through such "shell" corporations. The MCEBC sells bonds to the public. The bonds are repaid with revenue generated by the institution (ticket sales in the case of a football stadium or patient fees in the case of a hospital). The corporation then leases the building back to the Medical Center for thirty years, at which point the building then belongs to the Medical Center. "We started small to get exposure in the bond market," Melohn said.

The Guyton building was the first to be built with bonds sold by the corporation. The $14.5 million in construction costs were repaid with grant overhead, or the money attached to every grant for research earmarked for facilities expenses. The corporation was immediately successful in selling its bonds, primarily because Nelson had earned the Medical Center the reputation for strict fiscal management. Howard McMillan, who was president of Deposit Guaranty Bank at the time of Nelson's retirement in 1994, said, "The perception in the financial community is that the Medical Center is extremely well run and managed from a fiscal point of view, and Dr. Nelson's leadership has certainly been a major factor in that perception." But the Guyton building was only the test market for the Medical Center's entry into the bond market. What Nelson really envisioned was a way to finance the building of an entirely new hospital. That vision will become a reality with the completion of the newest hospital, the flagship University Hospital. At its occupancy, all the original hospital beds will have been replaced. But first would come the Blair E. Batson Hospital for Children, finished in 1997, named for the first chairman of the Department of Pediatrics, and later the Winfred L. Wiser Hospital for Women and Infants, the realization of the perinatal center long advocated by Nelson and Wiser. Donations through the Children's Miracle Network and the Friends of Children's Hospital helped pay for the Batson Hospital. The Wiser Hospital was entirely paid for with tax-exempt bonds issued through the MCEBC.

Before he retired in 1994, Nelson and Conerly had laid the groundwork for construction and renovation projects totaling $214 million. Only the expansion of the School of Nursing and the new construction for the School of Health Related Professions were paid for with appropriated funds. The others were paid for with tax-exempt bonds through the MCEBC or by self-generated revenues. The student union building, completed in 1999, the first building on campus devoted entirely to student activities, had been on the Medical Center's wish list virtually since 1955. The only place students had to meet outside the library or the cafeteria was a windowless room in the basement of the original building with a pool table and television. Student business was conducted out of whatever space was available. Not having a place where students could gather fostered a fragmentation of the student body. Nelson, thinking about how to finance the building, was astounded at the amount of money leaving the Medical Center in vending machines owned by the outside vendors. He replaced all the vending machines owned by outside vendors with ones the Medical Center owned and discovered an important revenue source for the student union. At his retirement, the IHL board approved the Medical Center's request to name the student union for him.

For as much building as he initiated, Nelson appreciated the natural beauty of the campus and its large wooded, park-like areas. It was one of the things that appealed to him when he came in 1973. The campus wasn't locked in by a concrete jungle as most urban health sciences campuses were. Marjorie Solomon said that Nelson cringed with every tree that had to be cut down for new buildings, but didn't allow his personal preferences to override his commitment to the future of the center.

Remaking the physical plant, a huge undertaking, was just the background noise for other events on campus. During the 1980s, the campus experienced a crime wave—a kidnapping from the nursery in 1980, the murder of a patient in the intensive care unit in 1981, another kidnapping in 1982, and the murder of a faculty member and suicide of her boyfriend in 1984. In both kidnapping cases, police found the babies unharmed within two days. Both were taken from the nursery on the fourth floor of the round children's hospital where mothers and fathers were encouraged to visit their babies. The kidnappings led to much stricter visiting policies and closer scrutiny of people visiting the babies. Police believed the ICU murder was fueled by the illegal drug trade. The victim was in the ICU because his killers had failed in their first attempt. They finished the job as he lay helpless in his bed while terrified nurses looked on. Dr. Maxine Eakins was the first female urologist on the Medical Center faculty and one of only a few in the entire country. She may well have had the distinction of having been the only African American female urologist. Urology was then and is now a male dominated specialty. The Mississippi native was coming home after being out of state for many years pursuing her medical training. She had completed a residency at Ohio State University in Columbus and joined the faculty the previous July. On April 3, 1984, the boyfriend that she thought she had left behind came into her office on the second floor of the clinical sciences wing, shot her several times, then shot himself. She died less than an hour after the shooting from wounds to her chest and abdomen. All of these events put Medical Center officials on notice that the world was no longer a safe place, and even institutions devoted to the care and well-being of people were not off-limits to criminal activity.

In 1980, the Medical Center celebrated its twenty-fifth anniversary with forty-two of its original staff members. At its twenty-five-year mark, Nelson pointed to the 67.4 percent of medical school graduates who were practicing in Mississippi. Eighteen of the first twenty-one School of Dentistry graduates—the first class had finished in 1979—were practicing in Mississippi, and three were in postgraduate training programs. That same anniversary year, the Medical Center's first director and medical school dean, Dr. David Pankratz, died in Oxford at the age of eighty-one.

Some of the issues the Medical Center struggled with during the 1980s were state versions of national debates such as the turf battle between the specialties of plastic surgery and ear, nose, and throat surgery. Surgery department chairman Dr. James Hardy maintained that the ENT surgeons had repeatedly violated agreements between them and plastic surgeons on staff as to what procedures each would do. The ENT residents wanted to do more cosmetic procedures, which had traditionally been the domain of the plastic surgeons. It was a fight being played out across the country, and one candidate for the chief of the division of otolaryngology (ENT) declined the appointment but told Hardy, "You are an innocent bystander in a national struggle." The division chief, Dr. Myron Lockey, had resigned, and in 1980 the ENT residents and fifteen local ENT physicians threatened to sue the Medical Center, alleging that Hardy had cooperated with plastic surgeons to prohibit the center's ENT residents and teaching staff from performing facial plastic and reconstruction surgery. Nelson refused to give in to their demands, and all the residents left. In 1981, the division head appointment went to Dr. Winsor Morrison, formerly of the University of Tennessee in Memphis, who later recruited Dr. Vinod K. Anand. Anand became division director when Morrison retired. When Anand resigned, the board approved the Medical Center's request to elevate otolaryngology to departmental status with a new name and new director in 2001. Dr. Scott Stringer became chairman of the Department of Otolaryngology and Communicative Sciences. It was the last of the surgery divisions to become a department following anesthesiology, neurosurgery, orthopedic surgery, and ophthalmology.

The Medical Center also felt—if not the wrath—the hostility of animal rights activists during the 1980s. This, too, was a struggle that had a national scope, but activists here never engaged in the kind of terror activities that plagued more urban centers. In some academic research institutions, animals were set free, labs vandalized, and equipment and data destroyed. The debate locally was much more subdued, but Medical Center officials felt threatened by the increasing demands of animal lovers. In 1984, the city of Jackson stopped its practice of selling strays that ended up in the city's animal shelter to the Medical Center and to the veterinary school at Mississippi State University (MSU). The previous year, six hundred strays were sold at five dollars per animal to either the Medical Center or to MSU. But the Medical Center exerted pressure of its own, and the city council reenacted the ordinance that allowed the sales, much to the annoyance of the Mississippi Animal Rescue League and some other pet owners.

"We're not anti-research," Debra Boswell, director of the animal rescue league, was quoted in the local press, "but they should get their animals from other sources."

Animals bred for research, the solution proposed by Boswell, cost about four hundred dollars each, compared to the five dollars that strays cost. Medical Center officials said a $5 million grant from the National Institutes of Health was at stake if the Medical Center couldn't guarantee a necessary supply of animals. Medical Center officials pointed out both the Food and Drug Administration and the National Institutes of Health strictly regulated the care that research animals received. A failed inspection could shut down an entire research project. They also pointed out that all animals ended up the same way whether in the pound unclaimed or in a lab. Both were euthanized. In the end, it became impossible to get pound animals. They were mysteriously unavailable. The Medical Center scientists finally resorted to buying all their animals from out of state.

Dr. L. William Clem, who was appointed chairman of microbiology in 1979 at the retirement of longtime chairman Dr. Charles Randall, had nothing to fear from animal rights activists who never blinked an eye about the way pond-raised catfish were treated in the lab. Clem came from the University of Florida where he had studied the immune system in salt-water fish. In Mississippi, he took advantage of the abundance of pond-raised catfish—always available and plentiful. During his years as chairman, he attracted millions of dollars in grant funds for his research and is widely recognized for contributions in describing the evolutionary development of the immune system. He and his team studied the relationship between temperature and the immune system extensively. Along the way to understanding the human immune system, he found some things that were helpful to the Mississippi catfish industry in reducing catfish mortality before maturity.

Research in the 1980s really took flight, and Medical Center investigators proved they could compete with investigators across the country in attracting large grants. Herbert Langford, professor of medicine, was one of the principal investigators in the Hypertension, Detection, and Followup Program (HDFP). In 1980, he explained the landmark results of that multi-year, multi-center study that proved aggressive treatment of mild hypertension could significantly reduce death from heart attack and stroke. The study resolved the dilemma of clinicians who often didn't treat patients with mild hypertension, believing that they were better off without drugs that often had uncomfortable side effects. The HDFP was important in the surge in development of new drugs for hypertension.

In 1985, the National Heart Lung and Blood Institute of the National Institutes of Health (NIH) awarded the Medical Center $6.4 million for its participation in the Atherosclerosis Risk in Communities (ARIC) study. With Dr. Richard Hutchinson and Dr. Robert Watson as principal investigators, the eight-year study, with four clinical centers participating, was designed to enhance the findings of the famous Framingham Heart Study. That study, also funded by NIH, followed individuals in Framingham, Massachusetts, for many years to determine what factors put them at risk for heart disease. But Framingham was a predominantly Caucasian community, and NIH wanted to know if risk factors in African Americans were the same. In the ARIC study, Jackson was the only center to look at an all-black population. The data from ARIC, especially the data from the Medical Center, and the groundwork laid in patient recruitment and retention led NIH to fund the Jackson Heart Study in 1999 with contracts to three institutions—the Medical Center, Jackson State University, and Tougaloo College—totaling $32 million. As early as 1965, Langford and Watson recorded blood pressures of every high school student in Hinds County, and their results showed that black students had higher pressures. Langford was, in fact, one of the first scientists to notice that race made a difference in blood pressure and risk of heart disease. And it is one of Langford's former students, current vice chancellor Dr. Dan Jones, who is determined that whatever differences exist in person's response to risk factors, it won't translate to a difference in health care. One of the goals of his tenure as vice chancellor is to make the Medical Center an instrument in ending health disparities among racial groups.

In the Department of Physiology and Biophysics, the 1980s saw a proliferation of data about blood pressure control from a whole raft of young investigators, all students of the department chairman, Dr. Arthur Guyton. They were working on one of NIH's program project grants that NIH had begun funding in 1968. In 2004, even after the death of Guyton, "Cardiovascular Dynamics and Their Control" is still funded by NIH, the longest running grant in NIH history.

In the Department of Pharmacology and Toxicology, Dr. I. K. Ho, later to become chairman of the department, was quietly one of the busiest, most productive members of the faculty. He did landmark work on the toxicity of organophosphates, a class of chemicals found in commonly used pesticides and in the nerve gas sarin, best known for its 1995 release in a Tokyo subway by the Japanese cult Aum Shinrikyo. In the 1980s, he was also doing pivotal research on the neurochemical basis for tolerance to and physical dependence on barbiturates, opiods, and cocaine.

In anatomy, Dr. Ben Douglas, later to become assistant vice chancellor for graduate programs, was hard at work on finding the key to a particularly virulent form of hypertension that attacked women in pregnancy, or pre-eclampsia. He thought his study of the condition would lead to an understanding of what causes other kinds of hypertension. It didn't, but Douglas became such an authority on pre-eclampsia that he became president of the International Society for the Study of

Pathophysiology of Pregnancy. The world group was formed to investigate and exchange information about factors that may endanger the lives of mother and baby, including infectious diseases, pre-eclampsia, nutritional deficiencies, and genetic disorders. Pre-eclampsia is still the leading cause of maternal-fetal mortality worldwide.

In 1995, the journal *Behavior Therapy* ranked psychology training programs on research productivity, and based on the number of publications originating from the Division of Psychology in the Department of Psychiatry and Human Behavior, the Medical Center division ranked as the fifth most productive in the world. The judges based the ranking on papers published in the twelve most prominent behavioral journals from 1974 through 1994. The journal failed to recognize that papers originating from the Department of Veterans Affairs Medical Center were part of the Medical Center's training program, and had they counted those fifty-nine papers the Medical Center program would have ranked third internationally right behind the University of London.

Clinical services, and research on clinical problems, also expanded greatly in the 1980s. The Department of Obstetrics and Gynecology flowered under the leadership of Dr. Winfred Wiser. Medical students all around the country clamored to get a slot in the highly regarded ob-gyn residency program, and Wiser was twice named best program director by the American College of Obstetricians and Gynecologists. Dr. John Morrison and Dr. Jim Martin pioneered important studies that ultimately led to safer pregnancies for women with diabetes, risk for early labor, or sickle cell anemia. Dr. Bryan Cowan developed the department's *in vitro* fertilization program, and the first test-tube baby was born in 1986. Dr. William Bates attracted a lot of media attention when his research led him to the conclusion that many women who wanted to get pregnant needed only to gain ten pounds, that the fat they lost when severely restricting calorie intake also did away with estrogen reservoirs.

While the ob-gyn department was adding clinical services, it was taking away a training program that, at one time, had vast emotional appeal. In 1983, Wiser announced he would begin phasing out the nurse midwifery program, which had trained 285 professional nurse midwives since it began in the late 1960s. But Mississippi had only 50 nurse midwives, and 9 of those taught at the Medical Center. Wiser also pointed out that no midwives had had clinical training at the Medical Center since 1976 because the labor and delivery suites were too crowded with staff physicians and residents who had to use the cramped space. In reality, most physicians in Mississippi didn't like working with midwives, and the only work midwives could find was among Mississippi's rural poor. Nurse midwives were trained to manage normal deliveries in healthy women. Unfortunately, it was this population of the rural poor that had by far the greatest risk of a complicated pregnancy. One obstetrician was quoted in the local press as saying he wouldn't mind working with nurse midwives if they were a part of a team whose leader was a physician.

Matthew Martin of Conehatta was the state's first bone marrow transplant recipient in 1982. Dr. Joe Files and his team in hematology extracted the bone marrow from Martin's brother and gave it to Martin, who had aplastic anemia. The bone marrow transplant program now has its own floor in the critical care hospital with areas carefully designed to maintain the sterile atmosphere so essential in the procedure.

Beginning in 1968 when the first children's hospital opened, pediatrics grew in response to the demand for services and together with the developing pediatric subspecialties. Under the leadership of Dr. Blair E. Batson, who recruited an array of pediatrician specialists in surgery, cancer, digestive disorders, neurology, endocrinology, cardiology, and newborn care, the Department of Pediatrics became well known to the people of Mississippi. Dr. Phil Rhodes in newborn medicine did important work that led to better treatment of premature babies that had hyaline membrane disease. Dr. Jeanette Pullen developed the children's cancer program, which significantly enhanced the care that pediatric cancer patients received, especially those with leukemia. Pullen is still active in the Pediatric Oncology Group, the network of centers that treat and do research on cancer in children and helped develop one of the protocols now used routinely and successfully on leukemia patients. Dr. David Watson in pediatric cardiology and Dr. Bobby Heath in surgery diagnosed and treated many children with congenital heart defects. In 1985, the Medical Center began its participation in the Children's Miracle Network, a fundraising effort for the nation's nonprofit children's hospitals. The annual event has done much to raise funds and an awareness of medical services available to children at the Medical Center.

In 1983, the IHL board approved the Medical Center's request to establish a Division of Emergency Medicine in the Department of Medicine. The specialty of emergency medicine was rapidly growing in response to the demand for better trauma care nationwide. Dr. Harper Hellems, chairman of the Department of Medicine, recognized that a separate division would greatly enhance the chances of getting an approved residency program in emergency medicine. Dr. Robert Jorden, who had been director of emergency medicine at the Denver, Colorado, General Hospital, was appointed the first director of the division in 1984. In 1990, the

University Hospital felt the impact of an upsurge in trauma patients that happened simultaneously with a nursing shortage. The critical shortage of available beds led to several instances of "diversion" in the emergency department. When ambulances headed to the Medical Center had a patient who would eventually require a bed in a unit that was full, the Medical Center emergency department told the ambulance to take the patient to another hospital. This raised the hackles of administrators in other hospitals. One of them wrote to state senator Cy Rosenblatt, who said his "unofficial poll indicates that UMC is on bypass greater than 70 percent of the time." He also raised the suspicion of the Quorum management contract. "How can it be reconciled that the UMC hospital is on ambulance bypass the majority of the days of the month and is refusing to accept referrals from outside physicians, yet is run by a for-profit corporation showing a multimillion-dollar profit yearly?" The criticism implicit in the charge was based on the common, but erroneous assumption that funds appropriated by the state paid for the trauma care that indigent patients received. In essence, why does the university turn away any patient when the state gives them money to take care of them? ER visits had jumped from 51,265 in 1989 to 55,058 in 1990, and Nelson pointed out that University Hospital's budget was derived largely from self-generated revenues (only 7.5 percent came from appropriated funds). Any income in excess of budget requirements is used to meet special needs of the teaching hospital, for which there are no appropriated funds. Nelson also explained several initiatives that would enhance nurse recruitment and retention. Finally, he told the hospital's critics that the contract with Quorum had cost the Medical Center $690,514 for fiscal year 1989–1990, but that savings in the same year, because of the Quorum contract, saved the Medical Center $970,000.

In 1989, Dr. Robert Smith, chairman of the Department of Neurosurgery, spent several weeks in the Soviet Union studying a minimally invasive treatment that the Russians had perfected for treating brain aneurysms. In doing so, he planted the seeds that led to the Palaces of St. Petersburg exhibit in Jackson in 1996. Smith and Yuri Zubkov, a famous Russian neurosurgeon, became good friends and collaborators. When pharmacist Buck Stevens and Mississippi's first lady Pat Fordice began their project of getting medical supplies for St. Petersburg, they, too, met Zubkov, who knew all the curators of the big museums in St. Petersburg. Dr. Brent Harrison, chairman of the Department of Radiology, got General Electric to donate a CT scanner to one of the hospitals in St. Petersburg. The organization formed by Mrs. Fordice and Stevens, sent millions of dollars' worth of pharmaceutical supplies to St. Petersburg. Zubkov talked the museum curators into lending pieces from their collections to Mississippi, as a way of returning a favor. Zubkov, who spent a year at the Medical Center as a visiting professor, was later murdered in Russia. The Medical Center named its imaging center the Yuri Zubkov Imaging Center in dedication ceremonies in 1997.

Surgeons at the Medical Center revisited transplant surgery during the 1980s. Surgery department chair Dr. James Hardy and his team had followed the historic operations in 1962 and 1963 with another heart transplant and another lung transplant in 1969. But increasingly, Hardy came to see that more work on the problem of rejection would have to be done before transplants would ever be a serious clinical option. In the 1980s, more immunosuppressive drugs were available, and Hardy had a new transplant surgeon, Dr. Seshadri Raju, who had impeccable surgical skills. In 1982, Raju performed the first liver transplant in the southeastern United States on twenty-four-year-old W. C. White of Natchez. He died two weeks after his transplant. In 1986, Dr. Raju and Dr. Bobby Heath did the first heart transplant at the Medical Center since 1969 on Larry Graves of New Hebron. Graves lived to attend many of the transplant reunions in later years. In 1987, Raju led the team that performed a rare double-lung transplant on a twenty-nine-year-old woman from Isola, Kathy Marshall. Before her transplant, Marshall had a long history of lung disease characterized by infections, asthma, and pneumonia. After her successful operation, she lived for many years and faced what is, by far, the biggest challenge of transplantation—paying for the high cost of immunosuppressive drugs to keep the body from rejecting the organ.

In May of 1988, Congressman Floyd Spence of South Carolina received his double-lung transplant at the Medical Center. His was one of Raju's most stunning successes. Spence arrived at the Medical Center debilitated by his illness, in a wheelchair and dependent on oxygen for breath. Post transplant, he got married, won reelection to the House of Representatives, and lived many years free of disease. The same year Spence received his transplant, at the very height of renewed transplant activity, was the year Dr. Robert Rhodes was appointed chairman to succeed Hardy, who retired in 1987. It was unfortunate for Raju and for those who wanted to see the Medical Center regain its ascendancy in the world of transplantation. Rhodes was an able administrator, but his critics said he did not spend enough time in the operating room to run a surgery department. Rhodes, who was a student of health care delivery and cost containment, saw transplantation as a depletion of limited resources in manpower and facilities. Liver transplants, particularly, required intensive postoperative care at a time when the institution could ill afford it. As department chair, Rhodes would not support Raju's direction of the transplantation program. Rhodes also initiated a departmental practice plan that, in Raju's opinion, threatened his livelihood. Raju, thwarted and rebuffed, sued Rhodes. It was an ugly and bitter episode in the Medical Center's history. Rhodes resigned after serving as chairman only seven years. He won the suit, with the court siding with the argument that the chairperson has the final authority in matters of the department. But nobody won. Raju is still a member of the Medical Center's clinical faculty, and he has a lucrative practice in vascular surgery at another local hospital.

The other very serious issue that faced Nelson in the 1980s was the accusation of scientific fraud by a member of the Department of Physiology and Biophysics. Nelson, department chairman Dr. Arthur Guyton, and officials at the National Institutes of Health, the agency Guyton's department depended on for the continuation of its research, received anonymous letters pointing to papers by a member of the department that the writer believed contained fraudulent data. Nelson appointed a committee of scientists on the faculty to review the accusation and the results of an internal investigation that Guyton had begun shortly after he got the letters. The committee recommended that enough evidence existed to warrant an investigation by the NIH. In 1985, the agency determined that the faculty member had, indeed, fabricated data. The NIH barred him from receiving grant funds for research or from engaging in any NIH activity such as serving on study sections or advisory panels. Guyton and other department members were found not to have been complicit in the fraud.

Still, it was a difficult three years, and it did not end with the NIH report. The faculty member retaliated against the department by suing Guyton, whom he likewise charged with scientific misconduct. The suit was announced in March, just as the state legislature was about to honor Guyton for his long career and many contributions. Nobody seriously believed the accusations against this paragon of scientific integrity, and after due process by the NIH, Guyton's reputation remained intact. For Guyton, the ordeal was harrowing. Toward the end of it, he told someone he hadn't slept for two and a half years. The only fault anyone could find with Guyton was his reluctance to believe anyone was capable of scientific fraud. Science was such pure joy to him, such a reward in itself, that he really had no understanding of the pressure others might feel to make data look better than it was.

In 1994, at age sixty-five, Nelson retired. He said then that he had made "mortal enemies" during his twenty-one-year tenure, but they couldn't be found among the faculty. He did the nearly impossible in higher education. He gained the admiration and respect of faculty members in all schools in spite of budget restrictions, space limitations, and parking prohibitions—all no-win issues for administrators. There were several factors that led to such widespread appreciation. Nelson is a person of charisma and charm, affable even in disaster, institutional or personal. He suffered a severe stroke in 2000 that left him without speech but not without communication skills. Nelson, with great affability, simply wins people over and gets them on his side. He has a sense of humor that his faculty appreciated. He delighted in showing visitors to his office his copy of *Playboy* magazine, in Braille, probably the gift of Dr. Sam Johnson, chairman of the Department of Ophthalmology. Johnson was probably the bearer of another gift Nelson cherished, a talking calculator designed for the visually impaired. He didn't need it for calculations, but took great pleasure in walking around campus pressing the square root function button over and over again. As he greeted colleagues in the hallways, "root, root, root" signaled his approach. He ended every annual faculty meeting with a joke, a practice that faculty began to think of as tradition.

Barbara Austin, director of the Division of Public Affairs since 1978, called Nelson "the fairest administrator" she has ever worked with. "He absolutely made decisions based on what was good for the institution even if that might be counter to what he wanted to do personally. And he was keenly aware that hardly any issue is all black or all white. He could see the gray. The Medical Center benefited enormously from his long tenure."

After a nationwide search, the IHL board approved the recommendation of Nelson's second in command, Dr. Wallace Conerly, as Nelson's successor. They were looking for a person who could take advantage of the momentum Nelson generated. Nelson left a robust and energized institution. A major building program was underway. Academic programs were strong; students in all the schools scored well above the national average in their professional exams. The Medical Center's endowment stood at $14 million, up from less than $200,000 in 1973. The board and the search committee agreed that the right person had been tapped. Former lieutenant governor Brad Dye, who worked with both Nelson and Conerly in legislative matters, said, "It was the most seamless transition I've ever known. I don't think the Medical Center missed a beat."

Conerly: Innovative Leadership

D r. Wallace Conerly had just begun his pulmonary medicine fellowship at the Medical Center in 1973 when Dr. Norman C. Nelson assumed the duties of vice chancellor for health affairs and dean of the School of Medicine. Six years later, Nelson appointed Conerly director of the Division of Continuing Health Professional Education when Dr. Roland B. Robertson left the Medical Center to be chief of staff at the Department of Veterans Affairs Medical Center.

Nelson had a keen appreciation of the importance of continuing education to the Medical Center. He had long since made it a separately functioning division with Robertson at the helm. Conerly impressed Nelson with his administration of the division, and Nelson named him assistant vice chancellor in 1981, moving him into his office suite. Nelson's previous assistant vice chancellor was Dr. David Wilson, the first director of University Hospital, who died the same year.

Thus began what was, in effect, Conerly's long apprenticeship in running the Medical Center. When Nelson began the program of campus expansion, he put Conerly in charge of overseeing new construction and renovation where Conerly excelled again. When Nelson retired in 1994 with construction projects still on the drawing board, it seemed only natural to leave it in the hands of the person who had a key role in developing the projects from day one. Conerly maintains he never had a clue he was being considered for the top post. Dr. Winfred L. Wiser, chairman of ob-gyn, chaired the search committee, and Conerly had submitted his name for consideration, but he thought the job would go to someone from outside the Medical Center.

"I had already told Chancellor [Gerald] Turner that I would be glad to stay around for a couple of years to help transition the new vice chancellor. When Dr. Nelson and the chancellor called me into Dr. Nelson's office to ask me if I would accept the job, I told them I'd have to think about it. It turned out to be a nine-year period I hadn't planned on."

Conerly's path to the Medical Center top office—Conerly says it's the equivalent of running a billion-dollar business—was as nontraditional as the internal succession. He did not, in his youth, desire to be a physician, and he did not, when he began medical training, start out with the intention of leading an academic health sciences center. Conerly grew up in Tylertown, Mississippi, a small town in Walthall County in the southwestern quadrant of the state. His father managed a hardware store in town, but the family moved to a farm in 1941. All during high school, Conerly, with two men his father hired to help him, managed the farm's two hundred dairy cows. They milked cows at 4 A.M. and again in the evening 365 days a year. The young dairy farmer had already been accepted at Mississippi State University where he was going to study animal husbandry. Conerly, fastidious in his personal habits and keenly attuned to the crooked lampshade in his office or the misplaced pen on his desk, remembers the precise moment that his career plans changed. "It was a cold, rainy morning before daylight in the winter of 1952. While I was milking, one of the cows swung her cold, wet tail right in my face. I decided farming might not be how I wanted to spend the rest of my life." Dairy farming never held any romance for him after that.

Conerly's two older brothers had gone to Millsaps College in Jackson, and Conerly followed their lead when it came time for him to choose a college. Two of his classmates were Eddie and Edna Khayat, older brother and sister to Robert Khayat, the future chancellor of the University of Mississippi. Conerly spent several weekends at their home in Moss Point never dreaming that his future and that of the high school youngster in the Khayat family would be so closely intertwined. In 1984, Khayat was named a vice chancellor of the university during the administration of Chancellor Gerald Turner while Conerly was assistant vice chancellor under Norman Nelson. "We spent a lot of time together working on different projects, and when Wally became vice chancellor and I soon thereafter became chancellor, I was tickled to death," Khayat said. "We had a healthy respect and affection for each other and worked together well. In all the years we worked together, there was never a cross word between us, even though we talked about a lot of touchy issues."

During his college years Conerly also met his future wife, Frances Bryan, in the chemistry lab where he was her lab instructor. They married after graduation. From Millsaps, Conerly went to medical school at Tulane University in New Orleans, graduating in 1960. He thought he wanted a career in the military and stayed in the air force for six years. He was a flight surgeon and worked with the astronauts of the Mercury program, including John Glenn and Scott Carpenter. Glenn seemed destined for selection even to the others in training. "While most of us were still eating breakfast, John Glenn would have already run ten miles," he recalled. "I worked with the original space program before there was a NASA. That was back when we would do the experiments on ourselves, on sensory deprivation, and the human centrifuge. There were fourteen of us vying for the manned orbiting laboratory."

It was his family that determined his decision to leave the air force. "I was enjoying myself tremendously. It was exciting and challenging. But I woke up and realized I had a son about to start school, and in the air force, if you're doing well, you're moving around." Even though he never went up as an astronaut, his familiarity with the Mercury and Apollo space programs and key players at NASA has been a major asset in the Medical Center's partnership with the agency.

The Conerlys moved to Jackson with their son, Al, and Conerly set up his general practice in south Jackson, developing relationships with the medical community that would last throughout his career. He says he actually made house calls, probably among the last of his generation to do so. His next career move was also decided by his family situation. "I loved private practice, but my practice grew to such an extent that I hardly ever saw my sons awake." By this time Frances had given birth to second son Charlie.

Conerly did a six-month fellowship at Ochsner's in New Orleans and then entered the internal medicine residency program at the Medical Center in 1971. From 1972 until 1974, he was the Mississippi Lung Association Fellow in Pulmonary Disease. He joined the Medical Center faculty in 1973. Conerly had no intention of staying in academic medicine but said, "I got hooked on teaching." During the next few years, Conerly was assistant (later associate) professor of medicine, while also serving as medical director of the Department of Respiratory Care in the School of Health Related Professions and as medical director of the adult intensive care unit, the acute care laboratory, and the hospital's respiratory therapy department and as director of Continuing Health Professional Education. Named assistant vice chancellor in 1981, he worked in the same office with Vice Chancellor Norman Nelson for thirteen years. "Dr. Nelson and I worked in the same office together every day as good friends and close associates. Dr. Nelson was a very successful leader, and I learned what he would do in nearly every situation. He moved out of his office his last day on the job, and I moved into it the next day. It was the most seamless transition imaginable."

Khayat points out that the practice of internal promotions—such as Conerly's and that of his successor Dr. Dan Jones—is often criticized by those who say an institution needs an injection of "new blood" to thrive and be creative in solving problems. Khayat agrees, but says the flip side is that much of the momentum of an institution's progress is halted by the steep learning curve a new person has to climb to be effective leaders in organizations as complex as both the Medical Center and the university. "I'm a real advocate of diversity and bringing new people into the system who've had a variety of educational experiences, but appointing someone to leadership who has an emotional investment in the organization and who knows the organization makes good sense, and I think it's proving to be a trend in higher education."

Conerly's nine-year tenure proved to be as atypical as his uncommon career trajectory. His leadership was marked by bold moves, sound business decisions, and new alliances that moved the Medical Center to unprecedented national prominence. Conerly was at his boldest in his decision to enter into the agreement that forged the Jackson Medical Mall Foundation. When the opportunity came to transform the old Jackson Mall into a health care center, Conerly admits that his main motivation was more space, not community improvement. The fifty-three-acre Jackson Mall, one mile west of the Medical Center on Woodrow Wilson Boulevard, was Mississippi's first shopping mall. It opened in 1969 when the area was home to many thriving businesses. By 1978, when Jackson's second mall, Metrocenter, opened in west Jackson on Highway 80, Woodrow Wilson and Bailey Avenue were no longer desirable business addresses. Customers increasingly chose Metrocenter over the Jackson Mall. In 1985, Northpark Mall in Ridgeland opened, catering to the increasing number of Jackson residents who had moved north to the rapidly expanding suburbs of Madison, Ridgeland, and the area around the Ross Barnett Reservoir. The Jackson Mall, once anchored by three large department stores— Gayfers, Woolco, and JC Penney—was in 1995 home only to Picadilly Cafeteria and a shoe repair shop. The largely vacant complex had become the target of vandals and a haven for crime.

Conerly credits Dr. Aaron Shirley for what the Jackson Medical Mall Thad Cochran Center has become—a model for health care delivery and urbran revitalization. "No project like the mall will succeed unless there is one person who has a passion for it. The Jackson Medical Mall succeeded because of Aaron Shirley's passion."

Shirley was the Medical Center's first African American resident and had been on the clinical (part-time) faculty in pediatrics since completing his residency. Shirley was director of the Jackson Hinds Comprehensive Health Center when the idea of using the mall as a health complex first occurred to him. At first he looked at space in the mall for a birthing center, but soon realized that if he could manage to carve out the four thousand square feet he needed for a birthing center, the rest of the mall was in such disrepair that it wouldn't be feasible. According to Shirley, Rueben Anderson, a former state supreme court judge, invited Shirley to meet him for lunch, and Shirley suggested they meet at Picadilly in the mall. Anderson wanted Shirley to serve on the board of directors of Tougaloo College, the private historically black college in Jackson. Shirley didn't really want to serve on another board. "I don't like boards, don't like meetings, and I told him I didn't think I was interested. He was insisting, and I was resisting. Finally, he asked, 'What would it take to get you to serve on the board?' Just off the top of my head, I said, 'Help me get this building. It would make a really nice health facility.'" Anderson, skeptical at first, agreed to find out who owned the building and how much they wanted for it. One of Anderson's law partners, Delbert Hoseman, is an expert tax lawyer who discovered that if Massachusetts Mutual Insurance Company, the mall owner, sold it to a nonprofit entity, they could use as a tax write-off the difference between the appraised value and what they sold it for. The Jackson Medical Mall Foundation would be the nonprofit buyer. "That was the first thing that made the deal possible," Conerly said.

About the time Shirley was eyeing the mall property and envisioning a future for it, Conerly and University Hospital director Ted Woodrell pondered the next move in housing outpatient services—the hospital's clinics that were so vital to the Medical Center's mission. Trends in health care were moving away from long hospital stays. In fact, more and more patient care was being delivered on an outpatient basis, in clinics. This trend alone warranted a new look at outpatient facilities. The hospital's clinics occupied nearly the same space they had in 1955, and more than 100,000 outpatients a year came to the 28,000 square-foot department. Those patients accounted for five hundred cars a day on the campus, creating congestion and often mayhem at the hospital's front door. In addition to the overcrowding, Conerly and Woodrell knew that if the Medical Center increased its outpatient numbers, which it could do only with more space, the Medical Center could maintain the number of hospitalized patients it needed for teaching.

Shirley said he and Ted Woodrell had been meeting every Tuesday morning almost from the time of Woodrell's arrival as hospital director. "We just talked about how the health center and the hospital could collaborate and just became friends," Shirley said. "I talked to Ted about the conversation between Reuben and me, and he agreed that it was something worth looking into."

Just before Norman Nelson retired, he had hired a firm to evaluate the hospital's future needs. In the plan for what became the new hospital construction on campus—the children's hospital, the women's hospital, the critical care hospital, and the new adult hospital—the consultants also pointed to the need for a free-standing 165,000 square-foot facility for outpatients and estimated that it would cost between $30 and $35 million. That report was delivered in 1994. It was the summer of 1995 when Anderson and Shirley met with Conerly to broach the subject of buying the mall. "Frankly, the only reason I listened to them at all was that report that was fresh on my mind. When they showed me the floor plan of the mall, I saw that the old Gayfer's store had 165,000 square feet, exactly the amount of space the consultants had said we needed for our clinics." The first partners in the mall plan were the Medical Center, the Jackson Hinds Comprehensive Health Center, the Mississippi Department of Health, and the city of Jackson. With the Medical Center's agreement to lease 165,000 square feet, it would be the "anchor" tenant. Moving quickly, Hoseman drew up the agreement that established the nonprofit Jackson Medical Mall Foundation. The founding partners, although they leased no space at first, were Jackson State University and Touglaoo College. The foundation purchased the mall for $2.7 million. The Medical Center's commitment to a fifteen-year lease at a cost of $1.2 million a year was the guarantee the banks needed to lend the money.

"I had a hard time selling the idea to the board," Conerly said. "I spent eight hours on the phone one weekend talking to individual [IHL] board members about the plan and finally convinced them." The board approved the Medical Center's leadership in the project in September 1995, and "we were up and running." The objections the board had to the project, said Conerly, were probably the same ones Conerly himself would have if someone had presented the idea to him.

"It had never been done before. It was a totally new concept, and none of the other institutions governed by the board had ever committed to such a lease. Just about everything about it was new, different, and untried. There were times when I thought maybe I was crazy, but I thought it was the right thing to do and pressed on. Had I known some of the opinions of the faculty, I may have had more second thoughts. Thank goodness I didn't know at the time. I chose not to consult with anyone about that decision. I don't know what that says about me, but I made most of the biggest decisions without consultation."

Sometime during the mall renovations, Shirley's organization, the Jackson Hinds Comprehensive Health Center, pulled out. "The board got cold feet, I think because they felt that their partnership with the Medical Center would diminish their standing. Without the health center, the foundation didn't meet the threshold of lease agreements required by the banks to guarantee the loan." With architectural plans already drawn, Shirley said, "I could see it, and I could taste it," and he didn't want to separate himself from it. He thinks, by then, Conerly was sold on the idea and didn't want the plan to falter, so when it was obvious the health center was not going to be a partner, Conerly stepped in and agreed to commit to more space to keep the financing on track. "This was a very painful time for me," Shirley recalled. His dream was being realized, and it was about to happen without him. But Conerly stepped in again and offered Shirley a faculty appointment in pediatrics so that Shirley could continue to play a role in the mall's development.

When renovations were completed and the Medical Center clinics opened formally on January 23, 1998, an official from the Department of Health and Human Services was enthusiastic about the mall's prospects. Doris Barnette, principal to the administrator of the Health Resources Services Administration, said, "When federal officials speak, they usually talk about shifting paradigms in health care. Believe me, you have shifted your paradigm here. Community-based care is a hot topic with health care planners. If someone in government doesn't know what that is, I can tell them where to find it—right here."

The Medical Center now leases 500,000 square feet of the total 800,000 available at the mall. The expanse of space and the direct access to the nearly 400,000 patients who use the clinics annually provide unique opportunities for innovative approaches to health care. The School of Pharmacy, for example, established the pharmaceutical care clinic where pharmacists teach patients to use equipment or take their medications. Physicians refer patients to the pharmacy clinic if they think the patient needs extra time in understanding how to use the treatments or medications prescribed for them. The Rowland Medical Library set up the Consumer Health Education Center where volunteers and library staff help patients search the Internet for information they or their families need or point them to printed materials available.

In setting up the Jackson Medical Mall Foundation, Conerly wanted Tougaloo College and Jackson State University as partners in anticipation of the three institutions working together on the Jackson Heart Study. The mall was neutral space where the three could collaborate on the first and largest study of its kind ever undertaken—the study of risk factors for heart disease in African Americans.

The mall foundation, in accordance with its governing rules, turned over a portion of its revenue from lease agreements to its three founding institutions on August 25, 2004. The foundation gave the Medical Center $2.5 million for an endowed professorship and $1 million each to Tougaloo and JSU. The foundation's seven-year pledge funds the Chair for the Study of Health Disparities at the Medical Center designated in honor of Aaron Shirley, now director of community health services at the Medical Center and chairman of the foundation's board of directors. Dr. Herman Taylor, professor of medicine and director and principal investigator of the Jackson Heart Study, is the first holder of the Shirley Chair.

While the mall project was probably the largest departure from University Hospital's traditional patient care mode, the hospital already had a presence fifty miles to the north of Jackson. Early in Conerly's tenure, just months after he had assumed the office in 1994, the community hospital in Durant in Holmes County was nearing closure. The state representative for that area, Mary Ann Stevens, appealed to Conerly for help in keeping the hospital open. As a result, the Medical Center entered into a lease agreement with the hospital and nursing home. The agreement allowed the people of Durant to keep their local hospital, and the University Hospital–operated emergency service gave the Medical Center another patient referral base. Six years later, in an outward movement Conerly didn't anticipate, Methodist Healthcare transferred ownership of its hospital in Lexington, also in Holmes County, to the Medical Center. The contract called for the transfer of $4,825,000 in assets and property to the Medical Center. The Lexington hospital, owned by Methodist since 1983, had eighty-four licensed beds and 160 employees at the time of the transfer. Conerly readily admits today that the rosy picture he painted in 2000 about the alliance with Lexington hardly told the complete story. "We didn't really want to take on another hospital, but the decision was forced on us by politics. We thought it would be a losing proposition, but when Methodist offered us the hospital, we couldn't really turn it down." Political leaders in the state house of representatives at the time promised the Medical Center that if it found itself in financial trouble with the hospital, state funds would be forthcoming. "Then the leadership in the House changed, and we got no such assurances."

The University Hospitals and Clinics was now a health care system with clinics at the mall and two hospitals and a nursing home in Holmes County. The geographical extension of the system necessitated changes in computer networks and transportation systems. The Jackson Medical Mall and all three units in Holmes County had to be linked to the main campus. The computer link came in 1997 under the direction of Dr. Roland B. Robertson who served as Conerly's assistant vice chancellor. One of his areas of responsibility was the upgrading of computer capabilities at the Medical Center, and in late 1997, a network linked all of the Medical Center's patient care areas. The same patient registration information could be accessed from the University Medical Pavilion, the clinic where physicians on faculty see their private patients, the Jackson Medical Mall and the hospitals in Holmes County.

Conerly made another bold decision that took the Medical Center not just across town and around the state, but to the highest echelons of the federal government. Conerly and university chancellor Robert Khayat knew a great many influential policy makers and politicians, but they decided they needed a more formal introduction to Washington. Conerly and Khayat hired the lobbying firm of Barbour

Griffith & Rogers, Inc., the "number one lobbying firm in Washington," according to Conerly. Its principals—Haley Barbour, now Mississippi's governor, former chairman of the National Republican Committee, Lanny Griffith, and Ed Rogers—had all worked together in the White House during the administration of President George H. W. Bush. "We just learned how Washington functioned and how to see the people we needed to talk to. We got to know the staff members, and we cultivated our relationships with Senators Thad Cochran and Trent Lott and Representatives Roger Wicker and Chip Pickering." Conerly estimates that the foray into the nation's capitol has resulted in some $40 million in appropriations to the Medical Center. "I don't think that's too bad," he said.

A special congressional appropriation of $12 million was one result of Conerly's careful cultivation of Washington contacts. It provided the start-up funds for the Medical Center's Cancer Institute at the Jackson Medical Mall, the goal of which is to have designation as a comprehensive cancer center by the National Cancer Institute of the National Institutes of Health within ten years.

In addition to the financial support garnered for the Medical Center from relationships in Washington, Conerly's close friendship with Cochran also resulted in a victory for animal research. In 2000, Cochran, at Conerly's request, introduced an amendment to an appropriations bill that prohibited the U.S. Department of Agriculture (USDA) from spending any of its appropriations on new regulatory measures. The USDA had agreed to a settlement with the animal rights group, Alternatives Research and Development Foundation (ARDF), that would have regulated the use of small animals—rats, mice, and birds—with as much vigor as larger animals are regulated. The settlement was viewed by the biomedical research community as "a surrender to animal rights extremists." The settlement would not have affected the Medical Center or other large research institutions where research is funded by federal grants. The small animals used at the Medical Center are just as vigorously regulated as large animals by the agencies that fund the research. What was at stake was the cost of doing research at the undergraduate level. Colleges all over the United States would have been hurt by the settlement that would have led to more red tape, more paperwork, and more inspections. "It was just a monkey wrench thrown into the nation's biomedical research effort," according to Dr. David Dzielak, associate vice chancellor for research at the Medical Center.

Much of Conerly's administration was characterized by extending the Medical Center beyond the confines of its North State Street–Woodrow Wilson location. "I saw the advantages of having the Medical Center become a more integral part of the community. Norman Nelson had concentrated on building up internally, and we had to do that. But the Medical Center needed to be more than the giant on the hill. We needed to become a visible part of the community." He credits his public affairs director Barbara Austin with planning and carrying out what he considered to be the key part in that plan. "Barbara planned monthly luncheons with leaders in every aspect of community life—state and city governments, law enforcement, religion, the arts, civic groups, health care, business, agriculture. A different group came every month, and I talked to them about the Medical Center, told them what we were planning, and explained how an academic health sciences center worked. In an informal and relaxed setting, we gave them an opportunity to know us better."

The institution's first attempt to bring in the public at large was the series of free public lectures by Medical Center faculty called MiniMed School. The first session was held in 1996 in a large classroom filled with people from the community. "We want to put a face on the Medical Center," Conerly said in the center's promotion of the series. "This is one way we can be good neighbors."

Base Pair is an outreach project that extends the Medical Center's resources to students in Jackson's public schools. The science mentoring program pairs high school science students from Jackson's public schools with a scientist at the Medical Center for an intensive experience in science—from lab work to making formal presentations of results. It started in 1992 and has received funding from the Howard Hughes Medical Institute since 1994. In 2002, the program, under the direction of Dr. Rob Rockhold, professor of pharmacology and toxicology, was recognized as a Role Model Institution by the national group, Minority Access, Inc. The group recognizes "exemplary practices in producing minority biomedical student researchers." Fifty percent of all Base Pair students have been African American. More than half the students in the program have chosen an undergraduate science major. Of those old enough to have graduated from college, 43 percent have entered graduate school and 37 percent are enrolled in a health care or science curriculum.

In 1998, Conerly asked the School of Nursing to help with the Work Ready Program of the Walker Foundation, a program that encourages welfare recipients to reenter the job force. Conerly asked Dr. Anne Peirce, then dean of the school, if her faculty could help by providing health assessments and screenings for the work-ready clients. It became evident to the nurses, however, that the midtown area residents needed more than episodic health care because they did not have access to affordable, quality health care. The result was the UNACARE Clinic, Mississippi's first urban health center staffed with nurse practitioners. It provides primary health care and education to residents of midtown Jackson, a community where a large portion of the population is medically under served.

One of the most innovative of the Medical Center's outward strategies during Conerly's tenure was the Telemergency program, developed as an answer to the growing numbers of rural hospitals without emergency care in 2002. Using telecommunications and medical imaging technology developed by NASA, physicians in the Medical Center's Department of Emergency Medicine communicate with nurse practitioners in rural hospitals throughout the state. Telemedicine is an emerging technology with few physicians willing to embrace it without reservation, but the Telemergency program illustrated an institutional commitment to solving some of the problems of access to health care in new ways.

As the Medical Center reached out during the Conerly years, it also bulged at the seams on its 164 acres. The major building program initiated by Norman Nelson was seeing its completion in the Conerly years. In 1996, two years into Conerly's administration, visitors looked up to see cranes and down into vast holes that would be the foundations for future buildings. Construction was ubiquitous with ten major projects underway on campus, including the Blair E. Batson Hospital for Children that would be occupied in 1997. While the Jackson Mall was undergoing its transformation, three groundbreaking ceremonies in 1996 marked the beginning of construction on the Winfred L. Wiser Hospital for Women and Infants, the Norman C. Nelson Student Union, and the new building for the School of Health Related Professions. The first of the ten projects completed was the expansion of the University Medical Pavilion, doubling the space where physicians see their private patients.

A real break in the perpetual parking impasse on campus came in November of 1996 with the opening of the first parking garage. Its 690 spaces doubled the number of parking places available to patients and visitors. Hospital director Ted Woodrell said it would "make a huge impact on our patients and their families."

On May 16, 1997, a dedication ceremony opened the eagerly awaited Batson Hospital, the first of four new hospitals to be built on campus. Three former patients participated in the ceremony that celebrated the victories of pediatric care at the Medical Center. Nina Washington, then sixteen, spent a month in the intensive care unit with congestive heart failure, a complication of lupus. She is now a medical student at the Medical Center. Chelsea Lanier of Vicksburg, then fourteen, spent months in the old children's hospital battling the effects of acute transverse myelitis. Andrew Carroll, then ten, had a heart transplant at the Medical Center when he was five. While the first children's hospital—the round addition on the south end of the adult hospital—was only thirty years old, the specialty of pediatrics had changed dramatically in that time. Patients with childhood cancer are often cured. New medications and antibiotics make the lives of cystic fibrosis patients infinitely better and longer. Pediatric neurology didn't even exist before the 1960s. And the flip side of this happy situation is that children have longer and more frequent hospital stays. Changes in treatment put increasing demands on physical facilities to keep pace. It was Blair Batson, the institution's first chairman of pediatrics, who pushed for the first children's hospital. Along with all his other contributions to the health of children in his more than three decades as chairman, he recognized that children—growing and changing by the minute—had very different needs than adult patients and needed their own space.

Dr. Owen B. Evans, Batson's successor in 1988, was equally committed to making the new hospital as suited to the twenty-first century as the old one was to its time. The small rooms in the old hospital, for example, were not designed for the monitors and specialized equipment used today. Nor were they designed for extended stays. Logistics for isolation were not considered because there was little need. AIDS did not exist, and neither did cancer survivors with medically suppressed immune systems. By contrast, the new hospital has rooms with separate air flow and ventilation to control the spread of infectious organisms. Each room has its own bathroom, and each room is large enough to accommodate a visiting parent comfortably. The entire hospital is designed in recognition of the unique needs of growing and developing children. Each floor has a play area with age-appropriate games and activities, and child-life specialists make sure that patients, even though ill and under treatment, have as many "real world" experiences as possible.

Evans holds the distinction of being the only pediatrician in Mississippi who is also a school superintendent. He's the head of the Batson Hospital School District, which has its own teachers who work with other teachers all over the state to help patients stay current with schoolwork. The same year the hospital opened, a $625,000 grant from the U.S. Department of Commerce allowed every room to be wired to the Internet to connect patients with friends and family, schools, or patients in other hospitals. The education coordinator for the hospital, Linda Shivers, hailed it as a great advancement in meeting the social development needs of hospitalized patients.

The cost of the $17 million building was borne in part by the people of Mississippi who contributed funds through the Children's Miracle Network and the Friends of Children's Hospital. In fact, the entire building is a testament to the generosity of Mississippians and to their support of the state's only hospital for children. The Mississippi Children's Cancer Clinic, the first floor of the Batson Hospital, opened in 1991. The Junior League of Jackson raised the funds to build the clinic, and at the time, it was the largest fundraising project any Junior League had ever undertaken.

As the clinic was being designed, Norman Nelson and Wallace Conerly insisted that the foundation be designed to accommodate future floors. With the help of funds made possible through the Children's Miracle Network and the Friends of Children's Hospital, the hospital added two additional floors for a pediatric surgical suite in 2004.

The second of the four hospitals in the Medical Center's long-range building program opened in 1999, the 160-bed Winfred L. Wiser Hospital for Women and Infants. Mississippi's only comprehensive hospital for women and infants, the $37.7 million facility is a six-story contemporary structure for women of every age and for newborns in the first few months of life. It is named for the obstetrics and gynecology department chairman who, in spite of cramped and outdated facilities, built one of the nation's premier ob-gyn departments. Winfred Wiser himself was a noted gynecologic surgeon, and he recruited physicians at the top of their respective fields to care for Mississippi's mothers and babies. The Medical Center, in fact, may be the only institution in the country to produce two presidents of the International Society for Maternal-Fetal Medicine—Dr. John Morrison, Wiser's successor as department chairman, and Dr. John Martin, professor of ob-gyn. Both made contributions to their specialty that changed the way doctors throughout the world deliver care to women with pregnancy complications. The neonatologists, or newborn specialists, matched the obstetricians in delivering excellent care in crowded facilities. More than 70 percent of the babies born at the Medical Center in any given year are at risk for dying or developing health problems. Their mothers need the specially trained maternal fetal medicine specialists who know how to prevent or deal with the worst complications of pregnancy, and the infants need the specialists in newborn care (neonatology) who are accustomed to saving even the tiniest babies with the most serious life-threatening conditions.

In the old newborn intensive care unit, on the fourth floor of the old children's hospital, the average patient count was seventy in a unit designed for a maximum of forty-two. Yet Dr. Phillip Rhodes, the director of newborn medicine, made a key discovery that changed the way premature newborns were treated at every center in the country. He found that supplemental oxygen delivered to babies whose lungs weren't mature enough to breathe on their own would actually damage lungs if given with too much force.

The third of the four hospitals opened in August of 2001—the critical care hospital. What had started as a two-story building for diagnostic radiology and a new medical intensive care unit turned into a stack of intensive care units. Conerly said he knew of no other hospital in the country exactly like it, but its placement and function make the delivery of critical care much more efficient at the Medical Center. It is connected both to the new adult hospital, to be finished in 2005, and to the emergency department and the adult surgical suites. The seven-story $23.5 million project houses offices for the Medical Center's helicopter crew, AirCare, on the seventh floor. The helicopter takes off and lands from the roof, one of the largest helipads in the country. Other floors hold the surgical ICU, neurology/neurosurgery ICU, a cardiac ICU, and a bone marrow transplant unit. At the building's dedication, Conerly noted, "We're able to buck national trends and realize this exciting expansion because of the tradition of fiscal conservatism here. We've saved for this and it's coming to fruition. No state money was used." In fact, of the entire $335 million building program, state appropriations were used only for the expansion of the Oglevee Building for the School of Nursing ($5 million), the new building for the School of Health Related Professions ($13.2 million), both completed in 1999, and the $4.1 million classroom addition targeted for completion in 2005.

After forty-four years without a student union, the Medical Center opened its first in 1999 and named it for Dr. Norman C. Nelson, vice chancellor for health affairs from 1973 to 1994. It was a fitting tribute to the man who always reminded his faculty and administrative staff that "none of us would have jobs if it weren't for students." Nelson set a high priority on meeting the needs of students first, so naming the union for him was met with unqualified support. At the dedication, the president of the Associated Student Body, Donnis Harrison, said Nelson wanted students to have a voice in their education and he listened to that voice. In the ceremony Nelson thanked the late chancellor Porter L. Fortune "for hiring me," Chancellor Gerald Turner, "who didn't fire me," and his wife, Annie Lee, "my best friend, my confidante and partner." The $9 million facility has a full-size basketball court; fitness facilities for aerobics and weight training; a walking track; a food court; meeting rooms for student groups; and a conference center for large meetings.

Looking at the construction boom on campus from the outside, a visitor would be hard pressed to imagine that the Medical Center was struggling with budget constraints. When Conerly addressed the faculty at the annual spring faculty meeting in 2001, he reported that after visiting the Department of Health and Human Services, federal officials had approved the upper payment limit of Medicaid reimbursements to the Medical Center, meaning that the institution qualified for the highest amount the federal health care payer would pay for services provided. He said it would mean an estimated $24 million in additional revenue each year for the Medical Center. Unfortunately, any gains in revenue from federal sources would be offset by the $21 million cut in appropriations from the state for the year beginning July 1, 2001. Still, hospital revenues were $23 million ahead of where they were at the same time the previous year, and grants from outside agencies were pouring in—$41 million at the time of the spring faculty meeting, twice the total for the year before and three times what it was six years previously.

By the fall faculty meeting of 2002, Conerly reported that "we've had two years of budget cuts." The Medical Center's operating budget went from $657 million in 2001 to $609 million in 2002. He credited the "thriving" hospitals and clinics for getting the Medical Center through the budget crisis. With patient numbers steadily rising upward with vastly improved facilities for delivering care, the hospital was indeed doing very well. In 1998, the University Hospitals and Clinics system was ranked number ten of the fifty fastest-growing American hospital systems. The research by Abendshien and Grube, a health care consulting firm in Northbrook, Illinois, examined net patient revenues between 1991 and 1996 of hospitals that had at least $100 million in revenues in 1996. The system recorded a five-year growth rate of 105 percent despite giving away $55 million in uncompensated care annually. That trend in hospital revenue continues, but the cost of providing uncompensated care has risen from $55 million to $100 million in 2004. The Medical Center defines uncompensated care as the services the hospital provides to patients who have no resources at all to pay for their care. Many hospitals define it as the difference between what an insurer pays for a service and what the hospital charges for the same service. If Medicaid, for example, pays for only a percentage of what a service costs, the Medical Center considers it paid.

A big jump in research funds also served to offset the budget cuts from the state. Conerly reported at the 2002 faculty meeting that research funding "has increased nearly four-fold, growing from $12 million in 1997 to more than $40 million in each of the last two years." Some of those large grants included $5 million to the School of Dentistry from the Partnership for a Healthy Mississippi to establish the ACT Center, a statewide tobacco cessation program directed by Dr. Karen Crews. The Partnership was created with the settlement Attorney General Mike Moore won for the state when he sued the tobacco companies.

The Institute of Neurological Disorders and Stroke of the National Institutes of Health awarded $3.5 million to Dr. Thomas Mosley in the Division of Geriatrics in the Department of Medicine to study changes in the small vessels of the brain. Mosley's theory is that small vessel changes lead to problems generally associated with the aging process and can be prevented by lifestyle changes in the same way that diet and exercise can help prevent artery occlusion leading to cardiovascular disease.

Dr. Andy Brown in the general medicine division of the Department of Medicine got a $4 million grant from the Department of Health and Human Services to develop a reproducible program that improves patient safety by reducing medical errors. A $9.4 million grant from the NIH established a Psychiatric Neuroscience Center in the Department of Psychiatry. The center trains the most promising young scientists to be tomorrow's brain scientists. They are taught by a highly talented cadre of neuroscientists recruited by former psychiatry department chair Dr. Angelos Halaris. The group studies the changes in the brain that occur in people with mental illness.

The enhancement of research had Conerly's full attention. He established the Office of Research, which for the first time in the institution's history, put all the mechanics of grant acquisition and research under one umbrella. He made $100,000 available annually to allow Medical Center scientists to apply for start-up funds for a research project. Large grants from federal granting agencies most often go to established investigators who already have good preliminary data. That makes it difficult for the scientist who's new to research to get established. A small grant for $10,000 or $20,000 can help a scientist do pilot studies or preliminary work that might be the basis for a much larger grant. He also established a program that gives monetary awards to scientists who are the most successful at bringing money into the Medical Center through research grants.

Both Norman Nelson and Wallace Conerly were adroit in their dealings with state lawmakers, and both genuinely appreciated the legislature's dilemma in not being able to fund all worthy state programs. Both knew that the Medical Center would have to develop new revenue streams for its major funding sources, and in 2002 state appropriations amounted to only 20 percent of the Medical Center's $579 million total budget. Back in 1962, the state had contributed more than half of the Medical Center's $5.8 million budget. As one of those outside revenue sources, the Medical Center's endowment increased significantly during Conerly's administration. Owing to the economic upturn in the early 1990s and the careful management of the funds, the endowment increased 93 percent in just six years, from $21.4 million in 1990 to $41.3 million in 1996. In 2001, the Medical Center raised $56 million in the university's Commitment to Excellence Campaign. As a whole, the University of Mississippi raised $525.9 million, more than twice the $200 million goal set by Chancellor Khayat. The Medical Center exceeded its $45 million goal by $11 million and increased its endowment to $82.1 million.

The Medical Center's clinical programs kept pace with the swiftly growing research enterprise. Two of Conerly's key appointments, both in 1998, were Dr. Rick deShazo as chairman of the Department of Medicine and Dr. William Turner as chairman of the Department of Surgery. Medicine is typically the largest clinical department of any medical school–teaching hospital, and Mississippi's is no exception. It trains the largest number of residents so, therefore, is responsible for a large portion of the services delivered in the University Hospital system. It is a critical department, and when Dr. Jack O'Connell filled the post in 1991, after Dr. Harper Hellems had retired, he began to move it from its languishing state. Hellems, who came in 1965, had been recruited by Vice Chancellor Robert Marston to succeed the first chair, Dr. Robert Snavely. Hellems retired in 1990, and although the department had grown in terms of numbers of faculty and research support, it wasn't keeping up with rapid changes in medical education. By the time O'Connell came in 1991, the department was having difficulty recruiting residents. O'Connell put some policies in place that began the process of change, but he resigned in 1996.

Dr. Rick deShazo came to the Medical Center from the University of South Alabama in Mobile where he was chairman of that Department of Medicine. With board certification in internal medicine, adult and pediatric allergy and immunology, rheumatology, and geriatrics, it is conceivable he could have gone anywhere. His acceptance of this key post really marked a turning point in the Medical Center's recruitment effort. DeShazo, like nearly every faculty member who's been recruited from out of state since the late 1990s, had only to look around him at the blossoming physical plant and reinvigoration of established programs to get a sense of the Medical Center's future. DeShazo saw the infinite potential for teaching and providing care that the Jackson Medical Mall represented. "In the past, internal medicine was almost totally hospital based. We had too little room to teach ambulatory care the way we wished. The space at the mall will give us a great opportunity to teach internal medicine the way it's practiced in the world away from academic medicine," deShazo said when he arrived on campus in January 1998.

After a national search, the IHL board approved Conerly's recommendation of Dr. William Turner to become chairman of surgery in 1998, succeeding Dr. Robert Rhodes, whose tenure as chairman was marked more by controversy than by progress. Turner, who was named the James D. Hardy Professor of Surgery, proved to be an excellent and energetic recruiter and rapidly filled the posts of directors in the department's divisions. Since his hiring, he has recruited sixty new faculty members to give the department a fresh scope and greater depth.

In 1998, the bone marrow transplant program was approved to perform unrelated bone marrow transplantation, meaning that patients at the Medical Center could now have a bone marrow transplant from a donor on the National Bone

Marrow Registry. In 2002, the unit received full accreditation from the Foundation for the Accreditation of Cellular Therapy the same month it moved into the new critical care hospital. Two hundred programs had applied for accreditation, but only forty-nine had received it in 2002. The diabetes center, located in the Jackson Medical Mall, was designed to be a comprehensive treatment center for patients with diabetes. In May 2001, the center's director, Dr. Marshall Bouldin, gave the press his "bad news, good news" take on the state of diabetes care in Mississippi. Based on parameters established by the Health Care Finance Administration (HCFA), the state of Mississippi ranked at the bottom in the way diabetes patients are cared for. "Mississippi has the worst record of any state for taking care of patients with diabetes," he said. The Medical Center diabetes team collaborated with the Mississippi Department of Health to form the new treatment center, and, based on the same HCFA parameters, the diabetes center at the Jackson Medical Mall scored better than the national average at providing diabetic care. Bouldin offered the concept as a boilerplate for other health care centers and hospitals to duplicate.

On November 13, 1997, friends and colleagues of Russian neurosurgeon Dr. Yuri Zubkov spoke at a ceremony that marked the opening of the Yuri Zubkov Imaging Center on campus. Zubkov, the chairman of the Department of Cerebrovascular Diseases at the A. L. Polenov Neurosurgical Institute of St. Petersburg, was murdered in Russia in February 1996. He was a man whose influence extended around the world, and the Medical Center in Jackson, Mississippi, continents away from St. Petersburg, was drawn into his orbit and was shaken at his sudden death. It was through his good will and influence that the museum curators of St. Petersburg allowed palace museum treasures to leave Russia for the first time and come to Mississippi for the Palaces of St. Petersburg exhibition. It was from him that Medical Center neurosurgeons learned new ways of doing surgery on the brain with balloon catheters. And it was Zubkov who was mourned by his Medical Center colleagues in a ceremony that was as much a memorial to Zubkov as a dedication of a building. But it is to those living that medicine attends, and the next day, the new interventional MRI was used for the first time to see and remove a brain tumor. The manufacturer of the new imaging-surgical tool, General Electric, chose the Medical Center as one of three original test sites for this revolutionary technology that would allow surgeons to see inside the body in nearly real time while they worked. Dr. Patrick Sewell used it for the first time in the treatment of lung cancer in July 1998. He threaded a probe to the lesions in the lung, guided by the nearly real time imaging, and froze two tumors that were causing the patient intense pain. In this case, Sewell was aiming for pain relief, not a cure, and it ended the patient's pain. In 1999, Sewell did the first cryosurgeries with the interventional MRI to remove tumors in the kidney. Three years later, none of the patients had recurrent kidney cancer at the treated sites, and none had lost kidney function as a result of having the procedure done. To patients with kidney cancer, this was good news indeed—a way to treat cancer in the kidney without having to remove the kidney. While removal of one kidney may not significantly interfere with one's life, the removal of a remaining kidney—the situation in which many kidney cancer patients find themselves—means a lifetime on dialysis. While the other two centers that had the interventional MRI—Harvard and Stanford—were still in the investigational stages with their units, the Medical Center was quickly putting it to clinical use. In addition to Sewell's procedures, Dr. Andrew Parent, chair of neurosurgery, and Dr. George Mandybur, associate professor of neurosurgery, were using it to reach and destroy previously inoperable brain tumors. Dr. Bryan Cowan, professor of ob-gyn, collaborated with Sewell on the successful trial of IMRI-guided cryosurgery for uterine fibroid tumors. NASA scientists saw the potential of IMRI-guided surgery for use on long space flights and teamed with Medical Center scientists, who rapidly became the world's experts in interventional surgery, to guide surgery in Japan—directed from the Medical Center.

Conerly had great vision, and he foresaw how important NASA could be to the Medical Center while the administration at NASA was looking for opportunities to use its technology for earth-bound research. One of the Medical Center/NASA collaborations has its origins in the computer model of the human body begun by the late Dr. Arthur Guyton and his former student Dr. Tom Coleman back in the 1970s. Over the years, Guyton and Coleman added massive amounts of data from work done by the scientists in the physiology department at the Medical Center. Dr. Richard Summers, professor of emergency medicine, was also a student of Guyton's and became proficient in building and running computer simulations. Now Summers, a physician, and Coleman, a research scientist, are using the computer models to help NASA deal with the detrimental effects of zero gravity on astronauts in the Medical Microgravity Project. After a prolonged period in a weightless environment, body fluids shift, and some astronauts have difficulty walking or experience dizziness when they reenter earth's atmosphere. A flight to Mars, which could take three years to reach, would be especially debilitating. Summers gathers physiological data from crew members before their space flight and again when they return to earth to add more data to the models.

At one point during Conerly's leadership, Medical Center faculty seemed particularly high profile on the national scene. In a January 2002 accounting, twenty-five members of the faculty led national medical and scientific organizations or edited prestigious medical and scientific journals. Dr. Ralph Vance, professor of medicine (oncology), was president-elect of the American Cancer Society. Others who held national offices included Dr. Rick deShazo, chairman of the Department of Medicine, president-elect of the Southern Society for Clinical Research; Dr. John Hall, chairman of physiology and biophysics, president of the American Physiological Society and the Inter-American Society of Hypertension; Dr. Rodney Meeks, professor of ob-gyn, president-elect of the Society of Gynecologic Surgeons; Dr. Steve Case, professor of biochemistry, president-elect of the National Academies of Sciences; Dr. Alan Freeland, professor of orthopedics, president-elect of the American Association of Hand Surgeons; Dr. James Martin, professor of ob-gyn, chairman of District VII of the American College of Obstetricians and Gynecologists; Dr. Larry McDaniel, professor of surgery (research), president of the Lancefield Society, a national organization devoted to the study of gram positive bacteria; Dr. Duane Haines, chairman of anatomy, president of the International Society for the History of the Neurosciences; Dr. Andrew Parent, chairman of neurosurgery, president of the Southern Neurosurgical Society; and Kit Stilley, associate professor of dental hygiene, immediate past president of Sigma Pi Alpha, national dental hygiene honor society.

While Conerly's tenure saw a robust and energized Medical Center emerging into national prominence, it was also a time of great loss. From 1996 through 2003, seventeen faculty members died, many of them from the ranks of the Medical Center's original faculty and staff. Dr. Forrest Hutchison, the center's first parisitologist, died in 1996. Lucy Lawson, microbiologist, appointed to the faculty in Oxford in 1950, and Dr. Orlando Andy, neurosurgeon since 1955, both died in 1997. Dr. Sam Johnson, first ophthalmologist and later chairman of the department, died in a rafting accident in 2000. Frank Zimmerman, the institution's first financial officer, died in 2001. Dr. Thomas M. (Peter) Blake, a member of the original faculty in the Department of Medicine, died in 2002. Dr. Arthur Guyton, first chairman of physiology and biophysics, as well as Dr. James D. Hardy, first chairman of surgery, died in 2003. Other deaths among the faculty included Dr. Ralph Carter, assistant professor of medicine, shot by a patient at the Department of Veterans Affairs Medical Center in 1997; Dr. Beth Hoskins, professor of pharmacology and toxicology, 1998; Dr. Nancy O'Neal Tatum, professor of family medicine, 1998; Dr. Harper Hellems, second chairman of medicine, 1999; Dr. Robert Blount, former dean of the medical school and Medical Center director, 2000; Dr. Patrick Lehan, cardiologist, 2002; Dr. Robert Smith, former chairman of neurosurgery, and Dr. Robert Currier, first chairman of neurology, 2003.

Dr. Bobby Heath, director of cardiothoracic surgery, drowned while scuba diving in 2000. During a trip to the People's Republic of China in 1997, Heath had taught Chinese surgeons how to do minimally invasive heart surgeries. Two million people in China need heart surgery mostly as a result of damage done by untreated streptococcal infections, and their surgeons wanted to learn the most cost-effective means possible to treat them. While Heath was there, he successfully did a coronary bypass on the father of one of the surgeons who invited him. Heath did all the pediatric heart surgery at the Medical Center and repaired faulty valves in the hearts of many Mississippi children. He was the transplant surgeon when children needed a donor heart. When the new class of medical students got their first white coats in a ceremony just days after Heath's death, Dr. Dan Jones, then the associate vice chancellor, told the students to conduct their lives and to practice medicine like Bobby Heath, to strive for self-confidence without arrogance. "He had all the self-confidence it takes to hold those baby hearts in his hands, but he was always Bobby from Duck Hill."

The national events that enveloped the Medical Center during Conerly's nine-year leadership included the preparation for potential computer crises with the beginning of the year 2000. With hundreds of computers used by employees and thousands of other computers imbedded in medical devices and monitors in every patient unit, the Medical Center, like other large institutions, began planning for Y2K four years in advance of the century change. On the eve of 2000, the Medical Center was staffed by key computer personnel, department heads, as well as the hospital personnel in patient care units. Except for a few minor computer glitches, the transition into the new century was a nonevent at the Medical Center. A practical joker dimmed the lights in the emergency room at the stroke of midnight causing a brief moment of panic among the ER crew, but otherwise it was business as usual on New Year's Eve in the emergency department.

Twenty-one months later, when passenger planes crashed into the twin towers of the World Trade Center building in New York City, the Medical Center became part of the national effort to combat terrorism. On September 12, Medical Center employees lined up to give blood, and in October, the Department of Medicine had three of its infectious disease specialists give a presentation on bioterrorism to a standing-room-only audience. Dr. George Taybos, associate professor of diagnostic sciences in the School of Dentistry, a member of the Mississippi National Guard, worked on the disaster mortuary operation response team with the Office of Emergency Preparedness in New York City in the aftermath of the attack. In August 2002, the Medical Center joined with six other leading research institutions and public health programs throughout the Southeast to form the Southeastern Center for Emerging Biologic Threats to combat biologic agents with potential for harm. The other founding institutions in the center are Emory University, the Georgia Institute of Technology, the Medical College of Georgia, the Morehouse School of Medicine, the University of Florida, and the University of Georgia. In December of 2002, in compliance with President George W. Bush's smallpox plan, the Medical Center offered the smallpox vaccine to three hundred Medical Center employees to form a smallpox response team if the variola virus were to be used as an agent of bioterrorism.

The university's hospital system, University Hospitals and Clinics, got the highest accreditation score in its history in 1999. The Joint Commission on the Accreditation of Health Care Organizations gave the system a high score of 90, putting it among the 25 percent of American hospitals that scored 90 or above. One site team visitor called it "the top one or two hospitals" she had ever surveyed. When the Southern Association of Colleges and Schools (SACS) made their visit to the Medical Center in 2000, the news was also good. At the fall faculty meeting just weeks before the SACS team came in October, Conerly had stressed the importance of the site visit to the entire institution. "Basically, without SACS accreditation, the Medical Center's other programs and schools can't get accredited." When the SACS team addressed the Medical Center at the exit conference, Dr. John Dwyer, associate executive director of the Commission on Colleges for SACS, asked the audience, "Do you know how this visit is different from all the rest? You have three commendations that came from this committee in its entirety. That's very rare. That's how you are different." The commendations, all entirely voluntary from the site team, were for the leadership "for its effective stewardship of financial resources," and for "its planning, construction and effective use of the physical facilities," and to the "administration, faculty and staff for their commitment to education and the general welfare of students." It was a resounding validation from an external source that the institution's commitment to excellence was not mere lip service.

The institution made an *A* on its report card, and Conerly got high marks personally from both houses of the Mississippi Legislature on "Conerly Day" at the state capital on March 19, just weeks from his official retirement date on June 30. Hundreds of well-wishers came to a reception in the capital rotunda, and both houses offered resolutions in praise of his service to the state. The hallmarks of his administration were enumerated: heightened national regard for the Medical Center, the attraction of record grants, a sharpened focus on research, development of the Jackson Medical Mall, tangible outreach to the community and to minorities, and unparalleled expansion of physical facilities. Conerly tells anyone who asks about his accomplishments that "it's all about relationships." In that, he excels. "Wally is an extremely likable person," said Chancellor Khayat. "He makes people feel comfortable, never condescending and never aggressive. And that 'good old country boy' way of talking doesn't fool many people." Khayat said in addition to the administrative skills Conerly possessed, "he was fully invested in this Medical Center—intellectually, emotionally, socially, physically—every aspect of his person was invested here, and it was to the Medical Center's great advantage." Conerly responded to the praise heaped on him on Conerly Day in his homespun characteristic vernacular whether he is in Tylertown, Mississippi, or in Washington, D.C. "My friend Heber Simmons gave me some good advice that I've tried to follow in whatever task I tried. He said, 'Wally, you should always leave the woodpile bigger than you found it.' I hope I've done that."

His successor, Dr. Dan Jones, noted that Conerly's leadership and decision-making style may appear unorthodox from a distance. "But close up, I see a remarkable instinct . . . based on solid values and principles. He does the right thing for the right reasons even when it may seem to put him at a disadvantage."

Jones came to the Medical Center in 1992 from Korea where he had run a hypertension clinic and taught medical students. Jack O'Connell persuaded him to come back and take up some of Dr. Herbert Langford's research projects. Langford, who led the Medical Center's participation in many national research studies on high blood pressure, died suddenly earlier in 1992. Langford had been Jones's mentor and had influenced his decision to specialize in the treatment of hypertension. Conerly picked Jones to be the chair of the medical school's curriculum committee because "we needed someone who was outstanding in terms of clinical skills and who also was a good researcher." In October of 1994, Conerly says the conversations began to start in earnest about what would become the Jackson Heart Study. "It was obvious to me that Dan was the right person to be the principal investigator of that because of his background in cardiovascular disease and hypertension and his recognized stature in the field." Conerly and Jones worked together very closely in putting together the Jackson Heart Study and both came to appreciate the other's talent. "He did an absolutely outstanding job," Conerly said. "He had the monumental task of getting people from all over the country to agree, the folks at the National Institutes of Health, the local community. It was huge project and it meant a lot to the Medical Center to get it. During that time, it became obvious to me that Dan would be the right person to take my job." Dr. Roland Robertson, who had been Conerly's associate vice chancellor, had removed himself from consideration when he announced his retirement.

Chancellor Khayat said he and Conerly, after talking about Jones as a candidate for vice chancellor, made a "quiet, national search" for other candidates. "We talked to several people, looked at resumés, and got some recommendations, but no one could top Dan's abilities. " Naming Jones associate vice chancellor would assure him an adequate apprenticeship.

Jones grew up in Vicksburg, went to Mississippi College, and graduated from the School of Medicine at the Medical Center. He completed his residency in internal medicine at the Medical Center and entered private practice in Laurel where his role model was Dr. Jimmy Waites, a graduate of the medical school class of 1958. From Laurel, he went to Korea. He says both he and Conerly had unorthodox training for leaders in academic medicine.

Jones took the helm of an institution that is ready to serve, and that is what Jones wants it to do. With many internal problems solved, the physical plant practically new, the Medical Center can tackle some of the big problems in health care. To Jones, the number-one problem is that good health is not equally divided among the races and economic classes. "The problem of disparity in health care is the biggest challenge we face, both in understanding it and how to fix it. We're addressing it in the students we select who will be the future health care providers. We want the ones with an interest in seeing the problem solved. We're addressing it in our research. The Jackson Heart Study represents the first time the medical establishment in this country has addressed the question of why African Americans are at higher risk for developing cardiovascular disease than their Caucasian counterparts."

While Jones has his own initiatives for the institution, he says it's important to stay focused on the Medical Center's key strength—its educational programs. "Excellence doesn't come automatically, but we have it now. All our educational programs are strong, and we have external validation for that both in test scores and accreditation reports. I would put our students against any student from any school in the country. As we mature and grow, we have to be careful not to lose sight of that."

It's no surprise that Khayat, having had a hand in picking Jones for his current job, is a big fan of the current vice chancellor. "My feeling is that the Medical Center will be stronger and stronger. Dan is a compassionate Christian and an astute administrator. He's going to lead this institution to greater levels of service, and I am a proponent of all his initiatives."

In seeking solutions to health disparities, Jones is simply refining what has been the goal of the Medical Center since its inception—finding ways to make life better for the state it serves through health care, the education of health professionals, and research. If all of those who conceived and birthed the Medical Center could see it at its fifty-year mark, it would be no surprise to them. They were all visionaries who dared to dream a huge dream—that a small medical center in a small, poor state would be a gleaming testament to humankind's quest to make life better for everyone.

CHAPTER 9

From One School to Five

The University of Mississippi Medical Center today is more than "the medical school" and more than "the hospital." The institution in its entirety includes four hospitals on campus and one in Lexington, and outpatient facilities (including the Cancer Institute) at the Jackson Medical Mall and in eleven other off-campus locations, known collectively as the University Hospitals and Clinics. It also includes five schools—medicine, nursing, health-related professions, dentistry, and graduate, all on the Jackson campus. The oldest of the five is medicine, established on the Oxford campus in 1903. Because its dean has always been the director or vice chancellor of the Medical Center, and because it was the medical school that moved to Jackson in 1955, its history has been related in the previous chapters. Each of the other schools, though inextricably intertwined with the development of the School of Medicine and the Medical Center, has its own history and course of development.

The School of Nursing is the second-oldest school at the Medical Center. The Mississippi Legislature, responding to reports that showed the need for more nurses, passed House Bill 291 in 1948 authorizing a Department of Nursing in the School of Medicine in Oxford that would be the state's first baccalaureate degree program for nursing students. The bill also made $60,000 available to equip the department and provide the personnel. The first chair of the department, Margaret Pinkerton, served only six months. The next chairperson, Christine Oglevee, stayed twenty-five years, moved with her department to Jackson in 1956, one year after the Medical Center opened, and became dean when the department was granted school status in 1958. Oglevee was the educational director for the Veterans Administration in Chicago before moving to Mississippi. "When I told my mother I was coming down here, she about had apoplexy," Oglevee was quoted as saying. "I told her I would either stay six months or the rest of my life." Oglevee had graduated from the Miami Valley Hospital School of Nursing in Dayton, Ohio, and had gone to the University of Chicago for both her BS and MS in nursing. When Pankratz, also a graduate of the University of Chicago, began looking for someone to direct nursing education in Mississippi, her name came up, and she came down.

Oglevee had the unenviable task of fighting the strong diploma nursing programs that were common throughout the state and were, in fact, the only other alternative to nursing education for students in Mississippi. "The diploma system amounted to the indenturing of nursing students," said Dr. Edrie George, who succeeded Oglevee as dean in 1974. The students worked long hours and were always assigned the evening and night shifts. The hospitals were reluctant to give up the programs because they were a source of free labor for them.

The dearth of large hospitals around the Oxford area presented a problem in finding sites where the first students—the three who enrolled in 1949—could get clinical training. The first students spent the first two years on the Oxford campus and two and a half years in selected hospitals. The first hospitals to provide clinical training were in Meridian, Greenwood, and Cincinnati, Ohio. The students enjoyed going to Cincinnati, but the mothers hated it, according to Oglevee. "I got calls day and night from parents." The Ohio placement didn't really help the state fulfill its nursing needs because many of the women met and married Ohio men.

The first class to enroll consisted of two "generic" students and one registered nurse (RN). Generic students is a term still used today that refers to students who've had no prior nursing training. Until 1964, students in each classification had separate undergraduate programs. In 1963, the National League for Nursing issued a directive to all baccalaureate schools that all students, generic or RN, be admitted to one undergraduate program. Inez Driskell was the first nurse in Mississippi to earn a baccalaureate degree from a Mississippi institution. She had a distinguished career as a public health nurse for twenty-seven years, and the Nursing Alumni Chapter of the University of Mississippi Alumni Association established the Inez Driskell Lecture Series to honor the memory of the school's first graduate.

Once on the Medical Center campus, student nurses took most of their clinical training in University Hospital, but they also rotated through the VA Hospital, the Department of Health clinics, the Mississippi State Hospital, and the Mississippi Sanatorium. While clinical training sites were plentiful, housing needs for other functions were not.

When Oglevee moved her students and faculty to the Medical Center in 1956, she did so knowing that they would have to share office and classroom space with the medical school until a building could be built just for nursing. The students, all female and all undergraduates, also needed a place to live because undergraduate female students were not allowed to live off campus unless they were living at home. The Medical Center leased an apartment building on Lakeland Drive for the students until the women's dorm was occupied in 1960. It wasn't until 1968 that female undergraduate students could live off campus. The first nursing education building, finished in 1963, was named the Christine Louise Oglevee Building in 1974, just weeks before her retirement in July. The most recent expansion and renovation of the building was completed in 1999.

In Jackson, the curriculum was shortened to four years from the previous four-and-a-half-year program. Students took the first year at any college or junior college they chose, then transferred to the Medical Center. At the end of the third year, students could be awarded a diploma and sit for licensure, or spend another year in preparation for the baccalaureate degree. In 1961, freshman nursing students were admitted to the Medical Center campus for the first time, which meant the school had to provide teachers for subjects such as history and English. That didn't change until 1975 under Edrie George's tenure. The school implemented the "two plus two" plan wherein students took core curriculum courses at any of the state's junior or senior colleges and transferred to the Medical Center for their junior and senior years. That curriculum remains in place today. "We didn't need to hire history teachers or English teachers. It wasn't cost-effective. Mississippi, along with Florida and California, has the strongest junior college system in the country, and we weren't using it. It saved the school the cost of hiring liberal arts teachers, and it saved the student's money if he or she took the first two years at a junior college."

George became dean in 1974 at the retirement of Dean Oglevee. George had earned the BS at the nursing school and knew Oglevee well. "She was a wonderful friend to students. We adored her. There was no problem you couldn't take to her." After George had been head nurse in the Medical Center's emergency room and a staff nurse in psychiatry, she went to graduate school at the University of Colorado for a master's in medical surgical nursing. She taught at Louisiana State University for a year before coming back to Jackson where Oglevee hired her to teach medical surgical nursing. She taught for four years, then got her PhD in education at the University of Mississippi. She taught in the nursing school for a year before she was appointed dean.

George, a reluctant candidate for dean, was urged by Vice Chancellor Norman Nelson and other faculty in the school to apply for the job. There were times during the first few years of her tenure she must have wished she had gone with her first instinct. By the late 1960s the state's demand for more nurses trained with graduate degrees had risen dramatically. In 1967, a second baccalaureate degree program in the state was open. By 1970, there were four baccalaureate programs, ten associate degree programs, and ten diploma schools. The Mississippi Nurses Association, the Mississippi State Medical Association, and the Mississippi Hospital Association all urged the establishment of a graduate program in nursing. The Board of Trustees of Institutions of Higher Learning mandated that all nursing faculty in all the state's nursing programs must have earned a master's degree by 1980, and in response to the demand, the Medical Center nursing school enrolled the first students in its master's degree program in 1971.

During George's first year as dean, the school had a scheduled visit from the National League for Nursing, the agency that grants nursing schools accreditation. As a result of the site visit, George said the League gave the school "reasonable assurance" of accreditation, pending the resolution of some recommendations made by the team of site visitors. But in 1975, the school received the bad news from the League: the graduate program was denied accreditation. Among the deficiencies noted by the League was an inadequate number of faculty with PhDs. George spent the next four years recruiting. At first, nurses with terminal degrees who wanted to come to Mississippi were few and far between. Then, toward the date set for the next site visit in 1979, "they seemed to come out of the woodwork," George said. By the time of the site visit, she had hired nine faculty with doctoral degrees, the other deficiencies were corrected, and the graduate program got full accreditation.

The undergraduate program has enjoyed continuing accreditation since its inception, and the master's program has been fully and continuously accredited since 1979.

The school established its own continuing education division in 1975, and that division sponsored the first Christine L. Oglevee Research Papers Day in 1980, two years after the death of the first dean. The division targeted the lay public for the first time in 1983 with its Woman's World program, a series of lectures and presentations devoted to women's health and other issues important to women.

George wrote the plan for the doctoral program in nursing that the IHL board approved in 1990. George retired that year, to be succeeded by Dr. Mary Ann Christ, who was dean from 1990 until 1995. The school's next dean, Dr. Anne Peirce, oversaw the significant increase in the school's research effort. The school began to play a major role in the research of the Jackson Heart Study by obtaining a grant to introduce nursing students from historically black colleges and universities to clinical research. And it was during Peirce's tenure that the nursing school received funds for its first endowed chair and the world's first endowed chair of nephrology nursing.

Dr. Kaye Bender became dean in 2003. Bender received both her undergraduate and graduate degrees in nursing at the Medical Center and rose through the ranks of the Mississippi Department of Health from public health nurse to deputy director. She holds a position unique to her predecessors in serving also as the

Medical Center's associate vice chancellor for nursing. Vice Chancellor Dr. Dan Jones made the appointment in 2004 "to give nursing a very strong voice in decision making" for the entire institution.

Throughout its history, the nursing school—with the state's first baccalaureate, master's program and its collaborative doctoral program with the University of Southern Mississippi—has pioneered nursing education in Mississippi.

The IHL board approved the establishment of the School of Allied Health on the Medical Center campus in 1971, and the school was operational in 1972. First known as the School of Allied Health, the Medical Center school was like many being developed across the country in response to the increasing need for standardization in the training of allied health professionals. As medical technology burgeoned after World War II, an increasing variety of highly specialized personnel became necessary to operate diagnostic tools, maintain hospital records, analyze the laboratory tests used in the diagnosis of disease, or direct a patient's rehabilitation. The training of these professionals had developed without a process whereby they could be standardized or accredited. The training often differed from one hospital to another and from one physician's practice to another. At the Medical Center, dental hygiene was funded through the vice chancellor's office; medical technology was housed in the Department of Clinical Laboratory Sciences; medical records was based in the hospital; and cytotechnology (the process of identifying cancerous cells in body tissue) was taught in pathology.

At first, the Medical Center's School of Health Related Professions assumed the administrative responsibility for the certificate programs in dental hygiene and medical record administration. Physical therapy was added in 1973 and became the school's first baccalaureate program. In 1976, respiratory care was added, and budgetary support for the medical technology training program was transferred to the school from the School of Medicine. The school added occupational therapy in 1978, assumed administration of cytotechnology in 1979, and added emergency medical technology in 1985. At one time, the curriculum included programs in nurse anesthesiology and in respiratory therapy.

The first dean, Dr. Thomas E. Freeland, arrived in July 1972 and in August requested that the IHL board change the name to the School of Health Related Professions. By 1973 work began on the refurbishing the men's dormitory for the school. It wasn't adequate space, and as the school added new programs and new faculty, additional space came from temporary buildings placed outside the dorm as well as leased and borrowed space around the area. Freeland came from California where he was deputy director of the allied health professions project in the Division of Vocational Education at the University of Southern California, Los Angeles. He was thirty-two at the time he was appointed dean and had earned the PhD at UCLA. His undergraduate degree came from Lock Haven State College in Pennsylvania and his master's degree from Long Beach State College in California. He came with primary interests in task analysis, work physiology, curriculum development, and manpower, and he brought with him his skill at writing successful grant applications. In 1974, the multi-million-dollar grant application he submitted to the Veterans Administration was funded, and the school began the highly successful State-wide Network of Allied Health Programs (SNAP). The seven-year funding period paid for a team of people to set up regional offices around the state and to make presentations at high schools, community colleges, and universities. Jim Baddley was the first director of SNAP, but he was hired by the Mississippi Hospital Association shortly thereafter. Jack Gordy, who had worked for the Mississippi Regional Medical Program, became the SNAP director and assistant dean of the school in 1976.

Members of the team included Ed King, David Allison, Patsy Hester, Linda Butler, and Cheryl Marble Windham. King retired from the school in 2004. Hester and Windam still work in the school. Gordy said they recorded as many as six thousand student contacts each year, promoting not just the school at the Medical Center but allied health programs throughout the state. "Our programs were necessarily limited in size, so there were always more students than we had room for. Our job was to increase the awareness of allied health throughout the state and to foster the development of allied health education." SNAP, in fact, was the springboard for the development of dental hygiene educational programs at Northeast, Meridian, Mississippi Delta, and Pearl River Community Colleges.

SNAP was so effective in building an awareness of allied health professions and the school, that the faculty continued to do the same activities that SNAP funded after the grant ran out.

One remarkable aspect of the school history has been its ability to respond quickly to health manpower needs of the state. No program is initiated unless there is documentation that a need exists for the graduates of that program. No student graduates from the school to find the market glutted with degree holders in his or her field. Gordy, who served twice as interim dean including one year before he retired in 2004, said the school kept up with health manpower needs through close association with the Mississippi Hospital Association and each of the allied health professional groups in the state. The nurse anesthesiology program was discontinued when the Medical Center's residency program in anesthesiology began to supply the state with enough physician anesthesiologists and because the nurse anesthesiology graduates were leaving the state to practice. The school discontinued its respiratory therapy program when community colleges began offering curricula that prepared ample numbers of qualified respiratory therapists.

The Medical Center's first computer network was in the School of Health Related Professions, according to Gordy. In the late seventies, Gordy and Freeland bought an early computer and began to do word processing on it. They soon realized that such school-wide projects as accreditation reports would be much easier to accomplish if all the faculty could access the report to make changes and corrections.

The school remains the only educational program on the campus that is physically removed from the Medical Center core, and early in its development, the physical separation caused problems. In a lengthy memo to Vice Chancellor Norman Nelson shortly after Nelson arrived on campus, Freeland's frustration was apparent. As he enumerated some of the problems in mail service, paging, and transportation, he also gave Nelson a detailed weather history of the past few months and noted the number of days on which there was significant rainfall. He urged a campus-wide courier system to transport items and mail from one side of the campus to the other.

Dr. Maury Mahan, who had been director of the Department of Institutional Research, was appointed dean in 1993 after the resignation of Freeland. The new building, finished in 1999, was completed during his tenure. It is connected to the old dormitory, which was renovated for faculty offices. Finally, all the school's educational programs are in one place. Only the anatomy lab, used for the dissection of cadavers, is housed away from the main building.

In terms of size, Gordy says there are certainly allied health schools that have much larger enrollments and many more programs. "We're right in the middle in terms of size." In terms of quality, Gordy points to the school's repeated victory in the nationwide competition for the Sydney Rodenberg Award given by Alpha Eta, a national honor society in allied health. The students compete with other students throughout the United States and are selected on the basis of academic achievement as well as the demonstration of leadership skills. "One of our students received the first such award ever given, and no other school has had as many students win it as we have."

Four of the school's programs offer the BS: clinical laboratory sciences (formerly medical technology), cytotechnology, dental hygiene, and health information management (formerly medical records technology). The occupational therapy program has been upgraded to prepare students for the master's of occupational therapy;

and the physical therapy program is phasing out its master's degree in physical therapy to offer the doctor of physical therapy degree. Occupational and physical therapy changes are reflective of the national trend toward higher degrees in these professions. The graduate degree program in the clinical health sciences, which is based in the school, prepares students who are already working as a health professional to earn master's or doctoral degrees. Students earn certificates in emergency medical technology.

Mahan resigned in 2003, succeeded by the current dean, Dr. Ben Mitchell, who was associate vice chancellor for institutional affairs at the Medical Center. Mitchell joined the Medical Center in 2001 when he left the Mississippi University for Women where he was vice president for finance and administration and professor of management information systems.

The Mississippi Legislature enabled the establishment of the School of Dentistry at the Medical Center in 1973 when it enacted House Bill 165. The law required the school to be operational within three years of the time funds were appropriated. The bill further stipulated that construction could not begin nor staff hired until Hinds County and the city of Jackson each contributed $1,250,000 toward construction.

Thus the school began with the unique distinction of being the only dental school in the country ever to have received construction funds from local governments. It would not be the last thing that set it apart. The first dean, Dr. Wallace V. Mann, was on board by January 1974. A graduate of Tufts School of Dentistry, he had specialized in periodontics at the University of Alabama and was on the Alabama faculty for eight years, ending his tenure there as chairman of periodontics and assistant dean. From Alabama he went to the University of Connecticut where he was chairman of the Department of General Dentistry and associate dean for graduate education. At the time of his appointment as dean, he was a consultant to the Council on Dental Education to the American Dental Association.

With the deadline imbedded in the legislation, the school had no time to dawdle. Eighteen months after the dean's arrival, in July 1975, the Medical Center broke ground for the dental education building. In August 1975, the first students enrolled. In August 1977, the building was complete. The first students had classes in borrowed space from the School of Health Related Professions and the nearby Mississippi Research and Development Center. One report had projected that it would take four years from the appointment of the dean to the admission of students. The dental school had done it in eighteen months.

There was yet another distinguishing characteristic of the school. Its "problem oriented" curriculum cut across disciplinary lines and was designed instead to teach the most common problems the student would encounter in a general dental practice. The school's graduates may elect to enter specialty training after four years in dental school, but if they chose not to, they would be ready to practice dentistry when they stepped off the stage after receiving their dental degree. Although it's been subjected to modification over the years, in 1995, Dean Perry McGinnis said, "The school still benefits from the organization of the curriculum."

After such an auspicious start, the school's almost universal approval would come to a crashing halt just nine years later. The Mississippi Dental Association (MDA) had lobbied the legislature in 1971 to create a dental school, and its members were among the school's most ardent supporters. In 1983, the MDA wanted the class size decreased. In 1982, the legislative Joint Committee on Performance Evaluation and Expenditure Review, known as the PEER Committee, issued a litany of complaints about the school ranging from accounting procedures to educational philosophy. It went so far as to recommend that if the school could not curtail its costs, the legislature should consider contracting with the Southern Region Education Board once again to educate the state's dentists by sending them out of state. Ironically, that had been one of the arguments for creating a dental school in state: when Mississippi students attended dental school out of state, they usually did not come back to Mississippi to practice. Medical Center officials thought that disgruntled members of the dental community had urged the PEER committee's report, and by 1985 the dental school-dental association relationship had become almost adversarial. It was the dental school's version of the town-gown problem that had almost derailed the medical school.

Another blow came in 1986 during one of the state's bleakest financial periods. Support for all higher education had been slashed. The IHL board, responding to the lack of funds, recommended that the School of Dentistry at the Medical Center, the College of Veterinary Medicine at Mississippi State University, Mississippi Valley University, and Mississippi University for Women all be closed. On the possibility of dental school closure, the MDA took a "no position" stance. If Dean Mann had any illusions about being able to please the MDA, they were dashed when an MDA committee wrote a letter to Chancellor Gerald Turner that concluded, "That spirit of cooperation between the academic and private sectors which is necessary for the existence of a quality school will be difficult if not impossible to redevelop with the current administration in place. While they did a magnificent job in starting the school, a different approach is needed if the

University of Mississippi School of Dentistry is to reach that full potential which is both possible and necessary for a quality institution." Mann had, in fact, already resigned to become dean of the University of Louisville School of Dentistry in Kentucky, a very significant career advancement to a highly qualified and distinguished dental educator. He later became the university's academic provost. Apparently his failings with the MDA didn't hurt his career. Mann died in 2004 after retiring from the University of Louisville.

Dr. John Hembree, whom Mann had recruited as chairman of restorative dentistry, became the school's second dean. Mann had hoped that Hembree's ties with the University of Tennessee, where many of Mississippi's practicing dentists had graduated, would help bridge the gap between school and profession. Hembree is a Memphis native who earned the dental degree from the University of Tennessee and had served on the faculty there from 1961 until 1978. He had been professor and chairman of the Department of Operative Dentistry of the College of Dental Medicine at the Medical University of South Carolina and associate dean for academic affairs and professor of restorative dentistry at the University of Detroit School of Dentistry.

The reluctant dean said he'd do the job for five years. It had all the earmarks of an impossible task. Morale at the school was at an all-time low. The cloud of possible closure frightened off a few faculty. Student applications slumped. Hembree, however, was an irrepressible optimist, and he was confident he could heal the breach with the practicing dentists. "I had gone to school with or taught half the dentists in Mississippi . . . and Wally [Mann] left me one heck of a legacy."

Less than a month after he became dean, Hembree mailed his first of a periodic newsletter to state dentists. He gave them example after example of reasons they had to be proud of the school: student GPAs (second only to Harvard dental school's entering class that year), national student awards, and 100 percent student participation in the American Student Dental Association. In the ensuing months he attended every state and district dental association board meeting in Mississippi, talking up the school and developing a nucleus of support. He met with the members of the MDA who had been critical of the school and listened to their concerns. The first long meeting dealt with thirty-seven issues. "Some were true; some were overstated; some were outright incorrect," Hembree recalled. He didn't flinch. He told them he would correct the valid complaints, and then he told them when each had been corrected.

With Hembree's commitment to communication with the state's dentists, the discord dissolved, and members of the MDA became the school's staunchest allies.

True to his word, Hembree resigned as dean after five and one-half years and returned to his research. He left the school strengthened and restored.

Dr. Perry McGinnis succeeded Hembree as dean in 1992 just in time to deal with yet another threat of closure. McGinnis joined the faculty in 1987 first as assistant then associate dean for academic programs. Like Hembree, he was a Tennessee grad who taught at UT from 1967 until 1977. McGinnis then went to Oral Roberts University where he was director and professor of oral pathology. No one fit the description of "a scholar and a gentleman" better than McGinnis.

The first signal that the dental school might be on the cutting block came early in 1992 with a Senate bill that proposed consolidating the state's universities. That bill failed, but later in the year, the IHL board, in a move to satisfy the courts in the Ayers Case (the desegregation class-action suit that had been dragging through the courts since 1975), again proposed closing the dental school, the vet school at Mississippi State, and Mississippi Valley University. This time it also proposed merging Mississippi University for Women with the University of Southern Mississippi, Alcorn University with Mississippi State, and Delta State University in Cleveland with the University of Mississippi. This time the MDA came out swinging in favor of "their" school, calling attention to "one of the best dental schools in the country."

Their claim was true. The dental school had flowered under McGinnis's gentle leadership. When the dean retired in 2001, a former president of the MDA recalled sitting in on an ethics seminar lead by McGinnis, and wrote this in tribute: "Gone was the fear and intimidation mode of dental education many of us remember. Replacing it was a new paradigm of trust, goodwill, and faculty-student sharing and interaction. In his position as teacher and dean, Perry has nurtured this educational model and is to be congratulated for its success."

In 1997, nine dental students were selected to present their research at the International Association for Dental Research. The school consistently has one of the highest percentage of its students represented in the national research forum. In 2000, the third-year students ranked fifth in the nation among forty-seven dental schools participating in the national board exams. In 2002, the seniors ranked sixth among fifty-two dental schools whose students took the national board exam.

Dr. Willie Hill, chairman of maxillofacial surgery in the school, took over as interim dean when McGinnis retired and spent a productive year at the helm. The school was in the middle of preparing for its next accreditation site visit. Results of that visit, received in August of 2003, were that all the school's programs were in "complete compliance" with all standards. Not only was it in full compliance, the site team singled out seven areas for special commendations. The school received special praise for its efforts in minority recruitment (17 percent enrollment of African Americans in the class entering in fall 2003), its strong research program, the strong level of state support for the school, the excellent basic science curriculum, the commitment to community health projects (part of the original curriculum hammered out by Mann and his first faculty), the program in clinical problem solving in general and the Grand Rounds program in particular, and the well-cared-for physical plant.

Dr. James Hupp succeeded Hill in 2002. Hupp holds the DMD (the doctor of dental medicine) from Harvard, the MD from the University of Connecticut, the JD from Rutgers University, and the MBA from Loyola University in Baltimore. He did his oral and maxillofacial surgery residency in the University of Connecticut and his residency in internal medicine at the University of California, Los Angeles. Before his appointment as dean of the dental school, Hupp had been assistant professor of oral and maxillofacial surgery at Vanderbilt, held joint appointments in the dental and medical schools at the University of Connecticut, was chairman of oral and maxillofacial surgery at the College of Medicine and Dentistry of New Jersey, and was chairman of oral and maxillofacial surgery at the University of Maryland.

One of Hupp's major changes in the structure of the school has been to appoint longtime members of the faculty to new leadership positions in the administration. In doing so, he acknowledges the rich heritage of the school as he moves it forward. Hupp inherited a very solid relationship with the practicing community, a relationship he hopes to continue with the establishment of a Board of Visitors. The group, made up of members of the community, including dentists, meets two or three times a year to discuss ways to link the school to the community. The bond between the MDA and the dental school couldn't be stronger. In 2003, all of the MDA's presidential officers were graduates of the dental school, for the first time in MDA history.

When the Medical Center opened in 1955, two graduates students joined the 135 medical students who enrolled for classes during the first registration. In 1959, the Medical Center awarded its first graduate degrees. Yet, until 2001, the graduate program at the Medical Center had been a part of the graduate school at the University of Mississippi. No individual at the Medical Center had even signed a diploma before 2002.

The graduate program was granted school status on July 1, 2001, and Dr. I. K. Ho was appointed dean of the School of Graduate Studies in the Health Sciences.

Ho has been chairman of the Department of Pharmacology and Toxicology since 1982 and was serving as interim associate vice chancellor for graduate studies.

Until 2001, graduate programs at the Medical Center were a loose confederacy administered by either the School of Medicine, Nursing, or Health Related Professions (HRP). Coordination between programs was difficult because medicine and dentistry are on the quarter system; nursing and health related professions on the semester system. If a student in HRP working toward a master's degree or PhD in clinical health sciences wanted to take a course in anatomy in the School of Medicine, converting credit hours was difficult. Now, all graduate students, with the exception of those enrolled in the master of science in nursing curriculum, are on the quarter system.

The school now offers twelve graduate programs—nine in the School of Medicine (the PhD programs in anatomy, biochemistry, microbiology, pathology, pharmacology and toxicology, physiology, and biophysics and preventive medicine, the MS in maternal-fetal medicine; and the master of biomedical sciences, professional portal track); one in the School of Nursing (the MSN and the PhD in nursing); one in the School of Health Related Professions (the MS and the PhD in clinical health sciences); and one in the School of Dentistry (the MS and the PhD in craniofacial and dental research).

In addition, the new MD-PhD program is administered by the graduate school. The option of receiving both the MD and the PhD has always been open to exceptional students, but it is now formalized to allow the student to get both degrees at the same time. Joey Bosarge of Pascagoula was the first student to complete the track and get the two degrees at the same time. Students who have been accepted into medical school and who are interested in pursuing a PhD as well are then invited to apply to graduate school. If their application is accepted, they complete the first two years of medical school, then enter a graduate program for three years, then take the third and fourth year of medical school. The Medical Center funds six students a year in the MD-PhD track, providing the Wallace Conerly Scholarship for medical tuition and a stipend to cover graduate school tuition—a total seven-year package worth $250,000. Ho says the program encourages clinician-scientists who understand both medical treatment and basic research.

Graduate degrees and the medical school have been interwoven for decades. The University of Mississippi awarded the first doctor of philosophy (PhD) in the basic medical sciences in 1950 to an anatomy student in the two-year medical school. Eighteen students in the two-year school earned the master of science (MS) degree in the basic medical sciences. The graduate program expanded beyond the medical school when six students received the Medical Center's first master of nursing degree in 1971.

In 1990, the IHL board approved the school's proposal to add the PhD in nursing in collaboration with the University of Southern Mississippi. The first students enrolled in HRP's graduate programs in clinical health sciences in 1995, and in 2004 the dental school enrolled its first graduate students. The master of biomedical science is a new two-year program designed to offer a master's degree suitable as preparation for teaching at the junior college level, as advanced training for governmental and industry positions and that will enhance a student's chances of gaining admission to medical, dental, and graduate school. Vice Chancellor Dan Jones publicly defended the program in an open letter to students and employees in the weekly Medical Center publication, *This Week at UMC*. A student, writing in the student newspaper *The Murmur*, criticized the administration's efforts to increase minority enrollment and mentioned the portal program in particular. Jones's letter made it clear that increasing minority enrollment in health professional education was crucial to ending health disparities, and that the portal program had his unqualified support.

Since 1955, when the Medical Center opened in Jackson, an individual at the Medical Center has been in charge of coordinating all the graduate programs, but the titles changed during the years. Dr. James C. Rice, chairman of the Department of Pharmacology and Toxicology from 1942 until 1959, served as chairman of graduate studies from 1955 until 1958. Dr. Charles C. Randall, chairman of the Department of Microbiology from 1957 until 1979, was appointed chairman of graduate studies in 1959. During his tenure, his title was changed to assistant dean of the School of Medicine in charge of graduate studies. Dr. W. Lane Williams, who was chairman of the Department of Anatomy from 1958 until 1979, was named chairman of the graduate council in 1968, a title that later changed to assistant vice chancellor. Dr. Ben Douglas, professor of anatomy, became the assistant vice chancellor for graduate studies when Williams retired, and when Douglas retired, Ho was named assistant vice chancellor. Vice Chancellor Wallace Conerly gave Ho the title of assistant vice chancellor for research and graduate programs to reflect two directives to Ho: to establish the Office of Research and to evaluate the need for an independent graduate school.

The graduate program's elevation to school status reflected its maturity and growth since 1955. With a record enrollment of 307 in 2004, up from 217 the year before, the school will never rival the enrollments in liberal arts graduate programs. "Graduate programs in the health professions are very nearly one-on-one in terms of faculty and students," Ho said. The structure and uniformity is now in place to enhance the curricula in each of the programs.

The new programs have a rich heritage of achievements earned by the older programs. The graduate faculty and their students have carried out some of the most significant research of the country's medical establishment. Microbiologists developed the pond-raised catfish as a model for studying the immune system. Physiologists at the Medical Center have made key discoveries of cardiovascular function that have defined the way physicians all over the world treat high blood pressure and congestive heart failure. Pharmacologists here are recognized around the world for their work in elucidating the mechanisms of drugs of addiction and environmental chemicals. A total of thirty of the Medical Center's PhD graduates in the basic medical sciences are department chairpersons all over the world. It could be argued that the Medical Center's graduate school, young in name only, is training scientists for the world.

Afterword

The University of Mississippi Medical Center today bears little resemblance to the Medical Center as it was in 1955. The original "T"—the medical school and the two wings of University Hospital—is barely discernible as the nucleus of today's sprawling physical plant. The medical school has been joined by the School of Nursing, the School of Health Related Professions, the School of Dentistry, and the School of Graduate Studies in the Health Sciences. The original University Hospital has been replaced by the Blair E. Batson Hospital for Children, the Winfred L. Wiser Hospital for Women and Infants, the Wallace Conerly Critical Care Hospital, and a new adult hospital to bear the flagship name of University Hospital. A major portion of the hospital's function is now carried out one mile west of the Medical Center at the Jackson Medical Mall Thad Cochran Center, the location of most of the Medical Center's outpatient services, including the Medical Center's Cancer Institute. In Holmes County, the Medical Center owns a sixty-bed nursing home in Durant and an eighty-four-bed hospital in Lexington.

From the first medical and graduate students who registered in 1955, enrollment in 2004 totaled 2,003 in all programs. From a faculty that numbered fewer than 50 in 1955, the total number of teachers in all schools is 776.

During the Medical Center's formative years, it depended on state appropriations almost entirely for its budget. Much of today's budget, well over $600 million, is self-generated or comes from other sources. Only 20 percent comes from state appropriations.

The Medical Center holds the promise of being one of the premier health sciences campuses in the country. Its physical plant is almost entirely new, and the sound financial practices of the past will pay dividends for a robust future.

The immediate future of the center is under the direction of the current vice chancellor, Dr. Daniel W. Jones. Jones has a long history in working with the nation's research establishment, the National Institutes of Health. He helped design the Jackson Heart Study, which has brought millions of dollars to the Jackson area. He believes the Medical Center is in a unique position to attract much more funding for clinical research. "Funding decisions are based on two things: need and the ability to do something about it. We have the need in Mississippi, and we've demonstrated a breadth and depth to our ability to address the need."

Jones sees the Medical Center as being ready, after years of building and gaining strength, to play a major role in eliminating some of the disparities in health care that exist in Mississippi. "That's the biggest challenge we face in health care today, and we're addressing it in the kinds of students we select, our research focus, and in the way we teach patient care."

Jones sees the mission of the Medical Center—teaching, patient care, research—as the instrument through which life can be made better for all Mississippians. That mission—through lean times and flush, through a succession of leaders and tremendous growth—hasn't changed in half a century.

Appendix 1

University of Mississippi Medical Center Institutional Heads

Dr. David S. Pankratz, 1955–1961, dean, School of Medicine and Medical Center director

Dr. Robert Q. Marston, 1961–1966, dean, School of Medicine, Medical Center director, and vice chancellor for health affairs

Dr. John Gronvall, 1966–1967, acting dean, School of Medicine and acting Center director

Dr. Robert Carter, 1967–1970, dean School of Medicine and Medical Center director

Dr. Robert E. Blount, 1970–1973, dean, School of Medicine and Medical Center director

Dr. Norman C. Nelson, 1973–1994, dean, School of Medicine and vice chancellor for health affairs

Dr. Wallace Conerly, 1994–2003, dean, School of Medicine and vice chancellor for health affairs

Dr. Daniel W. Jones, 2003–, dean, School of Medicine and vice chancellor for health affairs

Deans, School of Medicine

Dr. Waller S. Leathers, 1903–1924
Dr. Joseph Crider, 1924–1932
Dr. Philip S. Mull, 1932–1935
Dr. Billy S. Guyton, 1935–1944
Dr. James B. Looper, 1944–1946
Dr. David S. Pankratz, 1946–1961
Dr. Robert Q. Marston, 1961–1966
Dr. John Gronvall, 1966–1967 (acting dean)
Dr. Robert Carter, 1967–1970
Dr. Robert E. Blount, 1970–1973
Dr. Norman C. Nelson, 1973–1994
Dr. Wallace Conerly, 1994–2003
Dr. Daniel W. Jones, 2003–

Deans, School of Nursing

Christine L. Oglevee, 1948–1974
Dr. Edrie J. George, 1974–1989
Jeanette Waits, 1989 (acting dean)
Dr. Rene Reeb, 1989–1990 (acting dean)
Dr. Mary Ann Christ, 1990–1995
Dr. Rene Reeb, 1995–1996 (acting dean)
Dr. Anne Pierce, 1996–2002
Dr. Barbara Rogers, 2002–2003 (acting dean)
Dr. Kaye Bender, 2003–

Deans, School of Health Related Professions

Dr. Thomas E. Freeland, 1972–1993
Dr. J. Maurice Mahan, 1993–2003
Dr. Jack Gordy, 2003–2004 (acting dean)
Dr. Ben Mitchell, 2004–

Deans, School of Dentistry

Dr. Wallace V. Mann, 1974–1986
Dr. Harold Grupe, 1986–1987 (acting dean)
Dr. John Hembree, 1987–1992
Dr. J. Perry McGinnis, 1992–2001
Dr. Willie Hill, 2001–2002 (acting dean)
Dr. James Hupp, 2002–

Deans, School of Graduate Studies in the Health Sciences

Dr. I. K. Ho, 2001–

Appendix 2

Barnard/Guyton Distinguished Professors

The University of Mississippi Chancellor Gerald Turner established the Frederick A. P. Barnard Distinguished Professorships in 1988 on the Oxford campus and at the Medical Center. The recipients, each of whom receives a $10,000 cash award, are faculty members with a significant record of scholarly achievements and research. In 1998, Chancellor Robert Khayat changed the name of the professorships at the Medical Center to the Billy S. Guyton Distinguished Professorships to honor the memory of the medical school dean who played such a pivotal role in saving the medical school's accreditation and in assuring the future of the Medical Center.

University of Mississippi Medical Center Barnard Professors, 1988

Dr. L. William Clem, chairman, Department of Microbiology
Dr. Arthur C. Guyton, chairman, Department of Physiology and Biophysics*
Dr. Herbert G. Langford, Professor of Medicine*
Dr. Albert G. Wahba, chairman, Department of Biochemistry

University of Mississippi Medical Center Barnard Professors, 1993

Dr. L. William Clem, chairman, Department of Microbiology
Dr. John Hall, chairman, Department of Physiology and Biophysics
Dr. John Hembree, Professor of Restorative Dentistry
Dr. I. K. Ho, chairman, Department of Pharmacology and Toxicology
Dr. John Morrison, chairman, Department of Obstetrics and Gynecology
Dr. Jeanette Pullen, Professor of Pediatrics

Billy S. Guyton Distinguished Professors, 1998

Dr. Sandor Feldman, Professor of Pediatrics
Dr. John Hall, chairman, Department of Physiology and Biophysics
Dr. I. K. Ho, chairman, Department of Pharmacology and Toxicology
Dr. Michael King, Professor of Neurology
Dr. John Morrison, chairman, Department of Obstetrics and Gynecology

Billy S. Guyton Distinguished Professors, 2004

Dr. Julius Cruse, Professor of Pathology
Dr. Rick deShazo, chairman, Department of Medicine
Dr. Joey Granger, Professor of Physiology and Biophysics
Dr. Greg Ordway, Professor of Psychiatry (research)
Dr. S. H. Subramony, Professor of Neurology

*Deceased

Appendix 3

The School of Medicine gives the Waller S. Leathers Award, named for the first dean of the medical school, to the graduating student with the highest academic average over four years.

1957   Talbot G. McCormick Jr., Forest
1958   Walterine Herrington, Union
1959   Charles E. Sledge, Sunflower
1960   Charles Summers Mitchell Jr., Moss Point
1961   Robert Lange Elliott Jr., Greenville
1962   Walter Henry Rose, Moorhead
1963   Samuel Kimble Love, Itta Bena
1964   Frederick Ross Cobb, Inverness
1965   Julius Marvin Collum, Jackson
1966   James Wilson Aiken II, Senatobia
1967   James Douglas Brumfield, Jackson
1968   William Andre Causey, Jackson
1969   Thomas Lynn Windham, Jackson
1970   Jerry Clifford Griffin, Monticello
1971   Donald James Blackwell, Drew
1972   Mac Andrew Greganti, Merigold
1973   Stephen Hamilton Hindman, Newton
1974   Richard Evans Weddle, Eupora
1975   Donald Lee Roberts Jr., Long Beach
1976   Edward Harris Holmes, Clarksdale
1977   William Arthur Schmid Jr., Jackson
1978   James Ewell McDonald, Clinton
1979   James Robert Haltom, Natchez
1980   Richard Lavern Alexander III, Laurel
1981   Thomas Nichols Skelton, Jackson
1982   Hilton Lamar Gillespie Jr., Hattiesburg
1983   Charles Lamar Daley Jr., Jackson
1984   Allen Gafford Jones, New Albany
1985   Malcolm Sidney Moore, Tupelo
1986   Angela Dickson Graeber, Jackson
1987   Robert William Naef III, Jackson

1988 Daniel Paul Edney, Greenville
1989 Kevin Henderson Bond, Columbus
1990 James Rieves McAuley, Tupelo
1991 Steven Keith Rushing, Winona
1992 Celia Jenkins, Jackson
1993 Robert Towery McAuley, Tupelo
1994 Clay Broders Calcote, Jackson
1995 Lisa Kay Wooten, Ocean Springs
1996 Suzanne Ondine Dater, Jackson
1997 Bryan David Leatherman, Tupelo
1998 Curtis Lee Greer, Tupelo
1999 Alan Edward Jones, Jackson
2000 Richard Keith Johnson, Philadelphia
2001 Jason Arnold Craft, Brandon
2002 Kellan Elizabeth Ashley, New Albany
2003 Courtney McIntire Robbins, West Point
2004 Andrea Marie Furr, Houston

The School of Nursing faculty selects at least one student each year based on academic achievement and demonstrated leadership. In its first few years, there was only the faculty award, later named the Christine Oglevee Award in honor of the school's first dean. The Richard N. Graves Award honors the most outstanding registered nurse in the graduating class and may or may not be awarded each year.

1958 Jeanette Waits (Faculty Award)
1959 Mary Hellon Bramlett, Clarksdale
1960 Ann Pigford Hale, Sanatorium
1961 Guynell Strong Toney, Meadville
1962 Naomi Ruth Gilliam, Pascagoula
1963 Rebecca Cox Samuelson, Biloxi
1964 Nancy Carol Sigrest, Jackson
1965 Betty Earl Ross, Weir
1966 Dorothy Hall, Smithdale
1967 Theresa Goellner
1968 Harriet Drew Tucker, Hattiesburg
1969 Margaret Ann Valentine, Jackson
1970 Carol Ann Sitton McGehee, Jackson
1971 Cornelia Ann Armstrong, Tunica
1972 Sharon Elyse Greene, St. Petersburg, Florida
1973 Nancy Lois McCain, Petal (Faculty Award)
      Betty Jo Mulvihill Fedorak, Canton (Graves Award)

1974 Karen Mitchell Fly, Jackson (Faculty)
Je'anne Marie Barhonovich, Biloxi (Graves)

1975 Barbara Lee Hauser Prichard, Walnut Creek, California (Faculty)
Carol Hiersche LaCoss, Florence (Graves)

1976 Leslie Young Shands, Oxford (Faculty)
Doris Miniard Bryant, Pearl (Graves)

1977 Patricia Mary Draper, Maryville, New York (Faculty)
Virginia Lynn McKee, Merdian (Graves)

1978 Jenny Ruth Huntington, Wesson (Faculty)

1979 Kandi Kaye Korte, Metropolis, Illinois (Oglevee Award)

1980 James Adams Cheairs, Grenada (Oglevee)
Connie Lynn Lee, Picayune (Graves)

1981 Phyllis Gay Combs, Starkville (Oglevee)
Joan Purfeerst Williams, Brandon (Graves)

1982 Kathleen Severn Baer, Baton Rouge, Louisiana (Oglevee)
Merilyn Russell Charlton, Oxford (Graves)

1983 Wesley Morgan Madden, Forest (Oglevee)
Anita Kaye Bender, Laurel (Graves)

1984 Amy Mize Dudley, Jackson (Oglevee)

1985 Janie Lenton Clarke, Jackson (Oglevee)

1986 Kathy C. Walker, Jackson (Oglevee)

1987 Belinda Wellden Williams, Clinton (Oglevee)

1988 Janice Hill Clairain, Vicksburg (Oglevee)

1989 Beverly Elaine Fulgham, Mathiston (Oglevee)

1990 Loretta Cantrell Perry, Flora (Oglevee)
Deborah Tramel McCaffrey, Jackson (Graves)

1991 Amy Wallace Smith, Jackson (Oglevee)

1992 Rosmary Hale Dillard, New Albany (Oglevee)

1993 Kelly Caraway Boykin, Sandersville (Oglevee)

1994 Joynn Delle McLellan, West (Oglevee)
Betti Ann Blasi, Lauderdale (Graves)

1995 Lori Little Walker (Oglevee)
Wanda Newton Johnson (Graves)

1996 Michael Craig Robersohn, Jackson (Oglevee)
Charlotte Ann Godwin, Clinton (Graves)

1997 Shelia G. Bycofski, Clinton (Oglevee)
Harold Lee Dean, Meridian (Graves)

1998 Susan Guy Girani, Jackson (Oglevee)
Anne Elizabeth Berthold, Terry (Graves)

1999 Tommie Ann Kilpatrick, Isola (Oglevee)
Randall Ray Childres, Sanatorium (Graves)

2000 Glenn Alan Clark Gautier (Oglevee)
      Tracilia LaCole Brown, Jackson (Graves)
2001 Tara Nicole Price, McComb (Oglevee)
      Cynthia Aycock Roach, Madison (Graves)
2002 Gwendolyn Rene Mason, Walthall (Oglevee)
      Emma Carol Moran Parker, Pearl (Graves)
2003 Susan Dawn Inchcombe, Carthage (Oglevee)
      Carla M. Jones, Senatobia (Graves)
2004 Tina Denise McDyess, Shubuta (Oglevee)

The School of Health Related Professions gave its first award at graduation in 1980. The student chosen for the award was selected by fellow students. It was known simply as the Health Related Professions Award. In 1987, the school began giving the Virginia Stansel Tolbert Award to the student in the school with the highest academic average in the class for two years.

1980 Deborah Turner, Physical Therapy, Pascagoula
1981 Amy Hall, Dental Hygiene, Grenada
1982 Jeanne Marie Smith, Physical Therapy, Pascagoula
1983 Billie Fay Black, Dental Hygiene, Jackson
1984 Rachael Ann Williams, Physical Therapy, Newton
1985 Kimberly Dawn Freeman, Medical Record Administration
1986 Clara Bessie Ramos, Medical Technology, Jackson
1987 Kathryn Cecile Simmons, Dental Hygiene, Monticello
1988 Jennifer Lynn Pressley, Dental Hygiene, Coldwater
1989 Rebecca Lynn Henson, Physical Therapy, Weir
1990 Charles Michale Williamson, Physical Therapy, Prentiss
1991 Delma Ann Kinchen, Medical Record Administration, Picayune
1992 Mary Jordan Pitts, Physical Therapy, Indianola
1993 Bryant Wolfe Lary, Physical Therapy, Greenwood
1994 Kristine Kay Golden, Physical Therapy, Hattiesburg
1995 Daniel F. Bush, Cytotechnology, Long Beach
1996 Rachael DeLana Wade, Cytotechnology, Pascagoula
1997 Daniel Eric Crane, Occupational Therapy, Cleveland
1998 Jacqueline Ann Davis, Cytotechnology, Meridian
1999 Heather Renee Newlon, Physical Therapy, McComb
2000 Robin Milner Perry, Occupational Therapy, Vicksburg
2001 Jennifer Leslee Stokes, Occupational Therapy, Durant
2002 Amanda Carol Stokes, Occupational Therapy, Meridian
2003 Mary Patrice Sawardecker, Jackson
2004 Mara Carley Jepsen, Tupelo

The School of Dentistry has recognized the graduating student with the highest academic average over four years since the first class graduated in 1979. In 1987, the award was named the Wallace V. Mann Award to honor the school's first dean.

1979   John B. Smith Jr., Forest
1980   Alan Brooks Carr, Hattiesburg
1981   Hiram Alfonso Gatewood Jr., Raymond
1982   William David Simpson, Ripley
1983   James Edward Yelverton, Jackson
1984   Robert Scott Gatewood, Raymond
1985   Hugh Henry Rather, Holly Springs
1986   David Kennon Curtis, Brandon
1987   Marlon Dean Wakham, Drew
1988   Jeffrey Harold Brooks, Magee
1989   Anthony Kyle Chapman, Ocean Springs
1990   Jan O'Keefe Belote, Brandon
1991   William Thomas Neely III, Jackson
1992   Christa Irmgard Sligh, Ridgeland
1993   Jon David Holmes, Jackson
1994   Michael R. Nichols, Laurel
1995   James Strong Henderson III, Greenville
1996   Diana Sterling Tedder, McComb
1997   Sammy Dale Ellis, Walnut Grove
1998   Ivan Bryant Hirsberg, Clarksdale
1999   John Tracy Hodges, Tupelo
2000   Stevan Craig Fairburn, Hattiesburg
2001   Jennifer Gillian Ray, Clinton
2002   Paul Steven Arnold Jr., Natchez
2003   Richard Lee Simpson, Kosciusko
2004   Darren Keith Alexander, Gulfport

Sources

Chapter 1: **Our Island Home**

Bearss, Edwin C. *The Siege of Jackson.* Baltimore, Md.: Gateway Press, Inc., 1981.

Biennial Report of the Trustees and the Superintendent of the State Lunatic Asylum to the Legislature of Mississippi, 1900–1901. Holdings of the Mississippi Library Commission.

Dockery, David, III. "Windows into Mississippi's Geologica Past." Circular 6. Jackson: Office of Geology, Mississippi Department of Environmental Quality, 1997.

Harrell, Laura D. S. "Medical Services in Mississippi," in *A History of Mississippi,* vol. 2, ed. Richard Aubrey McLemore, 524–25. Hattiesburg: University and College Press of Mississippi, 1973.

Hughes, Dudley J. *Oil in the Deep South: A History of the Oil Business in Mississippi, Alabama, and Florida,* 1859–1945. Jackson: University Press of Mississippi, 1993.

McCain, William D. *The Story of Jackson: A History of the Capital of Mississippi,* 1821–1951. Vol. 1. J. F. Jackson, Miss.: Heyer Publishing Company, 1953.

Ragland, Lee. "Destruction Can Hinge on Nature's Mood." Jackson *Clarion-Ledger,* October 28, 1990.

Rowland, Dunbar. *History of Mississippi: The Heart of the South.* Vol. I, 599, 707–8. Chicago: S. J. Clarke, 1978; reprint of the 1925 edition.

Williams, Billy. Personal Interview. March 23, 2003.

Chapter 2: **Bilbo Medicine, Guyton Healing**

Bridgforth, Lucie Robertson. *Medical Education in Mississippi: A History of the School of Medicine.* Jackson: Medical Alumni Chapter and Guardian Society of the University of Mississippi Medical Center, 1984.

Brinson, Carroll, and Janis Quinn. *Arthur C. Guyton: His Life, His Family, His Achievements.* Jackson, Miss.: Oakdale Press, 1989.

Cruse, Julius. Personal Interview. March 28, 2003.

Fisher, William Bowlyne. "Contributions to Academic Medicine by Medical Certificate, M.D. and Ph.D. Degree Graduates of the University of Mississippi, 1903–1976." Doctoral dissertation submitted to the faculty of the University of Mississippi, August 1976.

Flexner, Abraham. *Medical Education in the United States and Canada: A Report to the Carnegie Foundation for the Advancement of Teaching.* Bulletin No. 4, 249–51. Boston: D. B. Updike, Merrymount Press, 1910. Reproduced by William F. Fell Co., 1960.

Guyton, Billy S. Correspondence from 1935 to 1936. Rowland Medical Library (RML) Archives, University of Mississippi Medical Center, Jackson.

Hardy, James D. *The World of Surgery, 1945–1984: Memoirs of One Participant.* Philadelphia: University of Pennsylvania Press, 1986.

Hardy, James D. Videotaped interview on February 21, 2002, for the RML Oral History Project, RML Archives, University of Mississippi Medical Center, Jackson.

Sansing, David G. The Billy S. Guyton History of Medicine Lecture, University of Mississippi Medical Center, 1995.

Sansing, David G. *The University of Mississippi: A Sesquicentennial History.* Jackson: University Press of Mississippi, 1999.

Chapter 3: **Years of Transition**

Annual Report of the Chancellor to the Board of Trustees of Institutions of Higher Learning for the period of July 1, 1955, through June 30, 1956.

Batson, Blair E. Personal Interview. July 30, 2003.

Bridgforth, Lucie Robertson. *Medical Education in Mississippi: A History of the School of Medicine.* Jackson: Medical Alumni Chapter and Guardian Society of the University of Mississippi Medical Center, 1984.

Brooks, Thomas M. Videotaped interview on December 7, 2001, for the RML Oral History Project, RML Archives, University of Mississippi Medical Center, Jackson.

Correspondence and documents compiled by Maurine Twiss, RML Archives, University of Mississippi Medical Center, Jackson.

Graham, Irene. Videotaped interview on December 11, 2002, for the RML Oral History Project, RML Archives, University of Mississippi Medical Center, Jackson.

Guyton, Arthur C. Speech given at the dedication of the David S. Pankratz Building, April 13, 1993.

Hardy, James D. *The Academic Surgeon: An Autobiography*. Mobile, Ala.: Magnolia Mansions Press, 2002.

Hardy, James D. *The World of Surgery, 1945–1985: Memoirs of One Participant*. Philadelphia: University of Pennsylvania Press, 1986.

Hilberman, Mark. "The Evolution of Intensive Care Units." *Critical Care Medicine* 3, 4, 1975.

Ludmerer, Kenneth M. *Time to Heal: American Medical Education from the Turn of the Century to the Era of Managed Care*. New York: Oxford University Press, 1999.

Neurosurgery News. A special issue dedicated to Dr. Orlando Joseph Andy, published by the Division of Public Affairs, University of Mississippi Medical Center, July 2001.

Program, Dedication of the David S. Pankratz Building, Division of Public Affairs. April 13, 1993.

Publication files, Division of Public Affairs, RML Archives, University of Mississippi Medical Center, Jackson.

Quinn, Janis M. "Lifetimes in Medicine." *Ole Miss Alumni Review* 44, 3, Fall 1995.

Quinn, Janis M. "UMC Presents New Hospital, Starts Another in Dual Ceremony." *This Week at UMC*, August 13, 2001.

Reiser, Joel. "The Intensive Care Unit: The Unfolding Ambiguities of Survival Therapy." *International Journal of Technology Assessment in Health Care*, Summer 1992.

School of Medicine Executive Faculty Minutes, 1948–1952.

School of Medicine Executive Faculty Minutes, 1953–1955.

Smith, Elvin E. "Recollection, Reminiscence, and Perspective on the Guyton Years at Mississippi." Unpublished manuscript, Department of Medical Physiology, Texas A & M University.

Stevens, Rosemary. *In Sickness and in Wealth: American Hospitals in the Twentieth Century*. Baltimore, Md.: Johns Hopkins University Press, 1989.

Twiss, Maurine. Conversations with Dr. Robert Currier, audio recorded on January 17, February 21, February 28, and June 6, 2001.

Waits, Jeanette. "The Nurses' Story," a brochure published by the Division of Public Affairs, University of Mississippi Medical Center, September 1995.

Chapter 4: **A Giant among Us**

Blotner, Joseph. *Faulkner: A Biography*. New York: Random House, 1974.

Brinson, Carol, and Janis Quinn. *Arthur C. Guyton: His Life, His Family, His Achievements*. Jackson, Miss.: Oakdale Press, 1989.

Guyton, Arthur C. "A Brief History of Cardiovascular Physiology at Mississippi." Manuscript in the Department of Physiology and Biophysics, University of Mississippi Medical Center, Jackson.

Guyton, Arthur C. "An Author's Philosophy of Physiology Textbook Writing." In *Advances in Physiology Education* 19, 1 (June 1998) in the *American Journal of Physiology Centennial*.

Guyton, Arthur C. Personal Interview. 1989. (date unknown)

Guyton, Arthur C. Videotaped interview on November 16, 2001, for the RML Oral History Project, Rowland Medical Library Archives, University of Mississippi Medical Center, Jackson.

Guyton, David L. Letter to Carroll Brinson, March 5, 1989

Quinn, Janis M. "Dignitaries Reach Conclusion: Arthur Guyton Rocks." *This Week at UMC*, November 20, 2000.

Quinn, Janis M. "Guyton Gets Nation's Top Medical Teaching Award." *This Week at UMC*, November 30, 1996.

Quinn, Janis M. "Guyton's Textbook, Number 10, Still Among Medical Best-sellers." *This Week at UMC*, September 22, 2000.

School of Medicine Executive Faculty Minutes, 1948–1952.

Taylor, Aubrey. Letter to the author, March 30, 1989.

Chapter 5: **Taking Down Barriers**

Associated Press. "Med Center's Mix Steps Please Feds." *Jackson Daily News*, May 29, 1965.

Author unknown. "UMC Welcomes Study of Mixing." *Jackson Daily News*, January 19, 1962.

Batson, Blair. Personal Interview. July 30, 2003.

Byers, Rowe. Personal Interview. March 30, 2004.

Coney, Ponjola. Personal Interview. January 27, 2004.

Ethridge, Tom. "State Men Listed among Signers of Petition Ignored by Congress." Mississippi Notebook. Jackson *Clarion-Ledger*, October 25, 1966.

Gordon, Bob. "'Youngster' Likes the Challenge as Med Center Head." *Jackson State-Times*, July 16, 1961.

Hardy, James D. *The Academic Surgeon: An Autobiography*. Mobile, Ala.: Magnolia Mansions Press, 2002.

Hardy, James D. *The World of Surgery, 1945–1985: Memoirs of One Participant*. Philadelphia: University of Pennsylvania Press, 1986.

Lasagna, Louis. "The Mind and Morality of the Doctor." *Yale Journal of Biology and Medicine*, April 1965.

Marston, Robert Q. Interviewed November 17, 1988, by Samuel Proctor for the Samuel Proctor Oral History Project of the University of Florida.

Oliver, James. Personal Interview. May 18, 2004.

Percy, Walker. "Mississippi: The Fallen Paradise," in *Signposts in a Strange Land*. Ed. Patrick Samway. New York: Picador USA Farrar Straus and Giroux, 1991.

Proctor, Jerry. "UMC Discovery 'Possibly' Biggest in State History." Jackson *State-Times*, January 19, 1961.

Quinn, Janis M. Brochure published by the Division of Public Affairs, University of Mississippi Medical Center, for the dedication of the Blair E. Batson Hospital for Children, May 16, 1997.

Sansing, David G. *Making Haste Slowly: The Troubled History of Higher Education in Mississippi*. Jackson: University Press of Mississippi, 1990.

Saxon, Wolfgang. "Robert Q. Marston, 76, Dies; Directed Institutes of Health." *New York Times*, March 16, 1999.

Shirley, Aaron. Personal Interview. August 27 and August 30, 2004.

Stevenson, H. L. "Legislators Halt Racial Integration." Jackson *Clarion-Ledger* (date unknown), 1956.

Toler, Kenneth. "Medical Center Drops Barriers." *Memphis Commercial Appeal*, May 29, 1965.

Twiss, Maurine. Unpublished interview with Robert Currier, April 11, May 2, May 9, May 23, and May 30, 2001.

United Press International. "Medical Center Planning CR Act Compliance." *Jackson Daily News*, February 23, 1965.

United Press International. "Race Mix Sought at UM Center." Jackson *Clarion-Ledger*, May 16, 1965.

Chapter 6: **Surgical Ascendancy**

Dalton, Martin L. "The First Lung Transplantation." *Annals of Thoracic Surgery* 60, 5 (November 1995): 1437–38.

Festle, Mary Jo. "First Try at a Second Chance: The Pioneering Lung Transplant." *Journal of Mississippi History* 64, 2 (Summer 2002).

Hardy, James D. *The Academic Surgeon: An Autobiography*. Mobile. Ala.: Magnolia Mansions Press, 2002.

Hardy, James D. "The First Lung (1963) and Heart (1964) Transplants in Man: Scientific Bases and Societal Dimensions in Retrospect." In *Jonathan E. Rhoads' Eightieth Birthday Symposium*. Philadelphia: J. B. Lippincott Co., 1989. Pp. 123–36.

Hardy, James D. *The World of Surgery 1945–1985: Memoirs of One Participant*. Philadelphia: University of Pennsylvania Press, 1986.

Hardy, James D. "Transplantation Vignettes from the Past." *The Chimera* 7, 3 (February 1997).

Hardy, James D. Videotaped interview on February 21, 2002, for the RML Oral History Project, RML Archives, University of Mississippi Medical Center, Jackson.

Hardy, Katherine. Personal Interview. June 6, 2004.

Keith, Virginia. Personal Interview. June 24, 2004.

McMullan, Martin. Personal Interview. May 25, 2004.

Ravdin, Isidore. Letter to James D. Hardy, November 15, 1957. James D. Hardy Memorial Library, Department of Surgery, University of Mississippi Medical Center, Jackson.

Surgical Forum, vol. 1. American College of Surgeons, W. B. Saunders, 1951.

Surgical Forum, vol. 34. American College of Surgeons, W. B. Saunders, 1983.

Thorwald, Jurgen. *The Patients*. New York: Harcourt Brace Jovanovich, Inc. 1971. English translation by Richard and Clara Winston.

Yelverton, Richard. Personal Interview. May 12, 2004.

Chapter 7: **The Nelson Years: Building Excellence**

Austin, Barbara. Personal Interview. September 1, 2004.

Coleman, Thomas. Personal Interview. April 20, 2004.

Conerly, Wallace. Personal Interview. May 4, 2004, September 7, 2004.

Dye, Brad. Personal Interview. June 5, 2004.

Hederman, Rea S. "Few Efforts Were Made to Satisfy HEW on Colleges." Jackson *Clarion-Ledger*, November 2, 1973.

Lovelace, Rupert. Remarks at retirement dinner for Norman C. Nelson, July 28, 1994.

Melohn, Brenda. Personal Interview. May 4, 2004.

Nelson, Norman C. Office files, RML Archives, University of Mississippi Medical Center, Jackson.

Quinn, Janis M. "The Good Doctor." *Ole Miss Alumni Review* 43, 2 (Summer 1994).

Reports from the University of Mississippi Medical Center submitted to the Board of Trustees, Institutions of Higher Learning, 1973 through 1994.

Soloman, Marjorie. Personal Interview. May 4, 2004.

United Press International. *Tupelo Daily Journal*, November 30, 1973.

Zimmerman, Martin. "Jackson Stops Sale of Stray Dogs for Medical Research." Jackson *Clarion-Ledger*, May 23, 1984.

Chapter 8: **Conerly: Innovative Leadership**

Coleman, Bruce. "$2.5 million JMMF Gift to Endow Shirley Chair at UMC." *This Week at UMC*, August 30, 2004.

Conerly, Wallace. Personal Interview. September 7, 2004.

Quinn, Janis M. "Accepting Massive Changes Like 'Kissing the Toad' for Princely Future Dividends." *This Week at UMC*, August 18, 1996.

Quinn, Janis M. "Anniversary Celebration at Durant Recalls 11th Hour Negotiations to Stop Closure." *This Week at UMC*, December 11, 1995.

Quinn, Janis M. "Biomedical Research Nationwide Gets Boost from UMC Action." *This Week at UMC*, October 16, 2000.

Quinn, Janis M. "Ceremony Marks Transition from Gayfer's to State-of-the-Art Clinics." *This Week at UMC*, February 2, 1998.

Quinn, Janis M. "Good Medicine." *Ole Miss Alumni Review*, April 2003.

Quinn, Janis M. "UMC Acquires the 84-bed Holmes County Hospital in Lexington." *This Week at UMC*, February 21, 2000.

Shirley, Aaron. Personal Interview. August 30, 2004.

Chapter 9: From One School to Five

Coleman, Bruce. "First Nursing School Dean Remembered at Reopening of Oglevee Building." *This Week at UMC*, October 11, 1999.

Coleman, Bruce. "Ho Appointed Dean of UMC's New Graduate School." *This Week at UMC*, July 30, 2001.

Coleman, Bruce. "Minority Nursing Students Hop Aboard the Jackson Heart TRAIN." *This Week at UMC*, August 14, 2000.

Coleman, Bruce. "Nursing School Gets First Endowed Chair with $1 Million Gift." *This Week at UMC*, July 5, 1999.

Coleman, Bruce. "Deputy State Health Officer Named Dean of Nursing." *This Week at UMC*, March 24, 2003.

"Dental School Establishes New Board of Visitors." *This Week at UMC*, February 23, 2004.

Fisher, William Bowlyne. "Contributions to Academic Medicine by Medical Certificate, M.D., and Ph.D. Degree Graduates of the University of Mississippi, 1903–1976." Doctoral dissertation, submitted to the faculty of the University of Mississippi, August 1976.

George, Edrie. Personal Interview. June 4, 2004.

Gordy, Jack. Personal Interview. October 19, 2004.

Ho, I. K. Personal Interview. October 25, 2004.

Myers, Leslie. "Hill Concludes Service as Dentistry's Interim Dean." *This Week at UMC*, June 10, 2002.

Myers, Leslie. "New SHRP Building a Model for Hands-on Allied Health Teaching." *This Week at UMC*, September 13, 1999.

Patton, Claudia. "At 25, SHRP's Enrollment Surge Coincides with Building Plans." *This Week at UMC*, November 13, 1995.

Program, *Christine L. Oglevee Research Papers Day*. Published by the Division of Public Affairs, April 19, 1980.

Quinn, Janis M. "Dental Survey Team Cites Seven Areas for Commendation." *This Week at UMC*, September 8, 2003.

Quinn, Janis M. "McGinnis Says Goodbye to Academic Dentistry at UMC." *This Week at UMC*, July 2, 2001.

Quinn, Janis M. "UMC Dental Students Put Efforts in Community Health." *This Week at UMC*, March 18, 1996.

Quinn, Janis M. "UMC Uses Tobacco Money to Curb Teen Smoking." *This Week at UMC*, October 25, 1999.

Reeb, Rene. *A History of the Graduate Program in Nursing*. Prepared for the 25th Anniversary Celebration, April 29, 1996. RML Archives, University of Mississippi Medical Center, Jackson.

Reeb, Rene. *The University of Mississippi School of Nursing, 1948–1991: A Chronology of Events*. Prepared as a special project for Dean Mary Ann Christ, 1991. RML Archives, University of Mississippi Medical Center, Jackson.

"School of Nursing Dean Named Associate Vice Chancellor for Nursing." *This Week at UMC*, July 5, 2004.

Twiss, Maurine. "History of the University of Mississippi School of Dentistry." Unpublished manuscript, Rowland Medical Library Archives, University of Mississippi Medical Center, Jackson.

"UMC Dental Grads Populate MDA in Historic Fashion." *This Week at UMC*, September 22, 2003.

Waits, Jeanette. *The First Quarter Century: A Brief History of the University of Mississippi School of Nursing, 1948–1973*. RML Archives, University of Mississippi Medical Center, Jackson.

Yelverton, Christie. "Hupp Named New Dean of UMC's Dental School." *This Week at UMC*, February 4, 2002.

Yelverton, Christie, "UMC Dental Students Rank Among the Nation's Best on Exams." *This Week at UMC*, September 25, 2000.

Yelverton, Christie. "UMC Faculty Member Helps in New York." *This Week at UMC*, October 22, 2001.

Index

Grenada, Miss., 19

Grenfell, Raymond, 47

Gronvall, John, 83–84, 89

Gulfport, Miss., 93

Guyton, Abraham Jenkins (grandfather of Billy), 22

Guyton, Arthur (son of Billy), 24, 27, 31–32, 34–35, 38, 43, 48, 57–78, 123, 127, 137, 145, 150, 171, 172; *Circulatory Physiology: Cardiac Output and Its Regulation*, 73; "A Concept of Negative Interstitial Pressure Based in Implanted Perforated Capsules," 74; death, 57; "Guytonian physiology," 57; "Physiological Syllabus," 70; polio, 24, 59, 63–65; Presidential Citation for the Development of Aids for Handicapped People, 65; *Textbook of Medical Physiology*, 43, 68, 70

Guyton, Billy Sylvester, 9, 14–24, 26, 50–51, 60, 62, 67; Guyton Clinic, 23

Guyton, David (son of Arthur), 63

Guyton, Greg (son of Arthur), 65

Guyton, Jack Smallwood (son of Billy), 60

Guyton, John Franklin, Jr. (brother to Billy), 22

Guyton, John Franklin, Sr. (father of Billy), 22, 23

Guyton, Joseph (father of John F., Sr.), 22

Guyton, Kate Smallwood (wife of Billy), 23, 60, 62

Guyton, Nathaniel (cousin to Joseph), 22

Guyton, Robert (son of Arthur), 65

Guyton, Ruth (née Weigle) (wife of Arthur), 34, 57, 62, 63–65

Guyton, Ruth Elizabeth (daughter of Billy), 60

Guyton, William Franklin (son of Billy), 60

Haines, Duane, 172

Halaris, Angelos, 168

Hall, John, 69, 74, 78, 172

Hall, R. W., 18

Hall, Yolanda Farkas, 94

Hand Surgeons, American Association of, 172

Harcourt Health Services, 70–71

Hardy, Bettie W., 120, 121

Hardy, Fred Henry (father), 99

Hardy, James D., 24, 27–28, 30–31, 35, 37–38, 40–41, 45, 46, 48, 50, 53, 81, 84, 99–122, 123, 126, 127, 137, 143, 149, 169, 172; *Academic Surgeon*, 53; *Hardy's Textbook of Surgery*, 126; *Pathophysiology in Surgery*, 105; *Surgery and the Endocrine System*, 103

Hardy, Julia (daughter), 120, 121

Hardy, Julia Poyner (mother), 99

Hardy, Julian (brother), 99–101

Hardy, Louise "Weezie" Scott Sams (wife), 34, 48, 102, 103, 104, 120–22

Hardy, Taylor (brother), 99

Hardy Society, 119

Hare, William, 28, 34, 48

Harper, Adolf, 95

Harrisburg, Pa., 101

Harrison, Brent, 148

Harrison, Donnis, 166

Harvard Medical School, 59, 64, 65, 120, 171, 188, 190

Hastings, Baird, 65–66, 73

Hattiesburg, Miss., 12, 42, 44, 93, 112

Head Start Program, 92

Health, Education, and Welfare, Department of, 87, 89, 90, 96, 132; Bureau of State Services, 98

Health and Human Services, Mississippi Department of, 26, 158–59, 166, 168, 180, 182

Health Care Finance Administration (HCFA), 170

Health Related Professions, UMC School of, 96–97, 123, 128, 135, 141, 155, 163, 166, 183, 186, 191–92, 195

Health Resources Service Administration, 159

Heath, Bobby, 147, 149, 173

Heidelburg Hotel, 33

Hellems, Harper, 128, 147, 169, 172

Hembree, John, 188–89

Hendrix, James, 105

Henry Ford Hospital, 60

Hernando, Miss., 94

Hester, Patsy, 184

Hibbing, Minn., 124

Hill, Willie, 189

Hill-Burton Act of 1946, 26, 28

Hilton, James, 48

Hilzheim, H., 3

Hinds County, Miss., 1, 26, 46, 186

Ho, I. K., 145, 190–93

Hoffman, Marie Louise, 35

Hogg, Ida D., 34

Holder, William E., 94

Holland, William, 87

Hollingsworth, Jeff, 118

Holmes, Verner, 50, 82, 89, 123, 125, 134, 138

Holmes County, Miss., 160, 195

Holyfield, H. N., 52–53

Hoseman, Delbert, 157

Hoskins, Beth, 172

Hospital Corporation of America (HCA), 10, 138–39, 148. *See also* Quorum Health Services

House Bill 165, Mississippi, 186

House Bill 291, Mississippi, 179

House Un-American Activities Commission, 94

Housestaff Association, 133

Houston, Miss., 19

Houston, Tex., 60

Howard, Billie, 71

Howard, Mary, 44

Howard Hughes Medical Institute, 162

Howard University Hospital, 93, 96

Hughes, Dudley J., *Oil in the Deep South: A History of the Oil Business in Mississippi, Alabama, and Florida, 1859-1945*, 6–7

Hughes, James L., 133

Hughes, Jerald, 42

Hume, Alfred, 11–14

Humphrey, Hubert, 86

Hunt, F. S., 3

Hunter, Carrie Paul, 92

Hupp, James, 190

Hutchinson, Richard, 144–45

Hutchison, Forrest, 172